"I have just finished your Chakra A
[text obscured]
to you enough how this has changed me for the better. I have a young child and problems with my ex-partner, and through your teachings you have helped me reconnect to myself. I no longer have anger, hatred, or negative thoughts. I can't wait to carry on this practice and make my mind, body, and soul stronger. I'm definitely trying to persuade friends and family to learn! Thanks for your help and time."

- Terri A., United Kingdom

"Thank you for the Chakra Awakening course. I appreciate Dr. Acharya Shree Yogeesh's kindness, compassion and generosity. Performing the chakra activation techniques and at the same time watching Acharya Shree's YouTube videos all seem to have a positive effect. I observed a general balancing and strengthening of my focus across the spectrum of my awareness and activities. I look forward to exploring the effects and perspectives over time."

-Henrik Y., United States

"The Chakra Awakening course is amazing. Even the Yogeesh Ashram YouTube channel is the best. For a real truth seeker the knowledge Acharya Shree Yogeesh is sharing is very precious and priceless. After repeatedly watching and listening to his videos, my attitude and understanding towards life has changed a lot. I totally believe that Siddhayatan is the heaven on this earth...Thank you is a very small phrase. Keep up your great work."

- Srikanthi B., United States

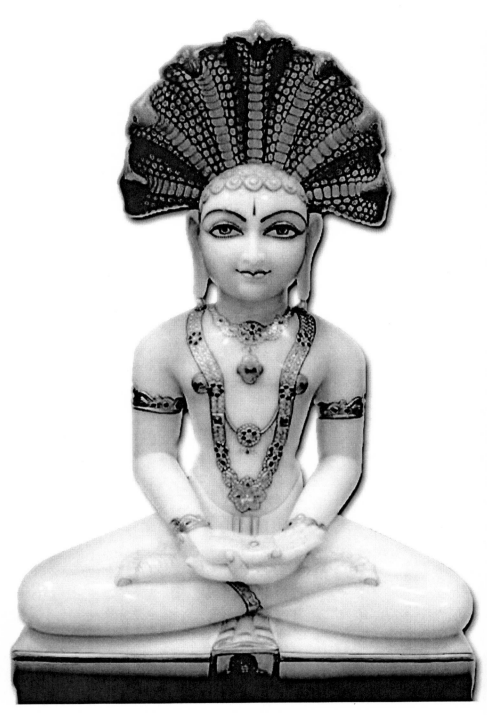

23rd Tirthankara Parshvanath
First Kundalini Master

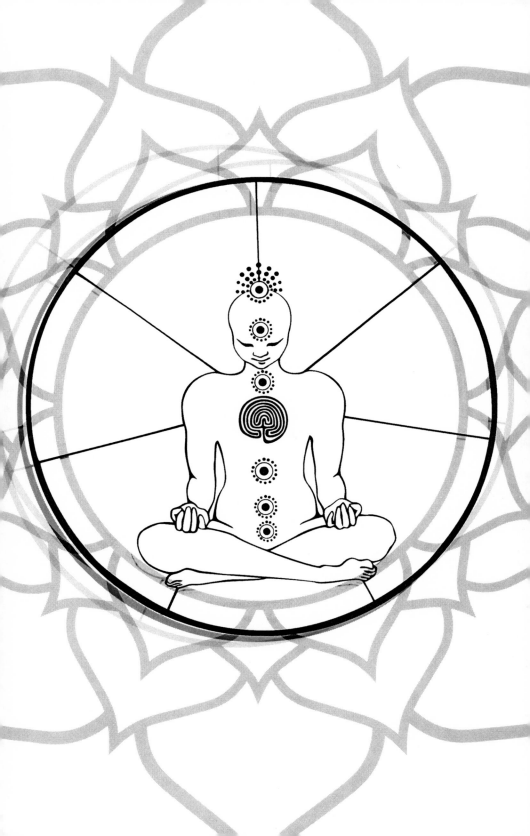

C H A K R A
A W A K E N I N G :
THE LOST TECHNIQUES

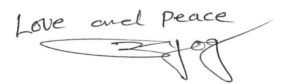

Love and peace

ACHARYA SHREE YOGEESH

Siddha Sangh Publications

SIDDHA SANGH PUBLICATIONS
9985 E. Hwy 56
Windom, Texas 75492
info@siddhayatan.org

Copyright © 2014 by Acharya Shree Yogeesh
Cover design: Rob Secades

www.siddhayatan.org
www.chakraawakeningbook.com

ISBN - 0-9843854-4-4
ISBN - 978-0-9843854-4-7

Library of Congress Control Number - 2014943251

Printed in the United States of America.

Disclaimer

Please note that not all exercises, diet plans, or other suggestions, mentioned in this book are suitable for everyone. This book is not intended to replace the need for consultation with medical doctors and other professionals. Before changing any diet, exercise routine, or any other plans discussed in this book, seek appropriate professional medical advice to ensure it is acceptable for you. The author and publisher are not responsible for any problems arising from the use or misuse of the information, materials, demonstrations or references provided in this book. Results are not guaranteed.

TABLE OF CONTENTS

FOREWORD

It takes courage to know the Truth. The moment you realize Truth is the exact same moment you realize something you thought to be True was a lie. Acharya Shree Yogeesh calls these moments "turning points" in one's life. You leave behind beliefs and realize and experience Truth for yourself. This is the path of spirituality. Nothing is new. Nothing needs to be discovered. But everything needs to be realized. It is all there, in you, if you know how to go beyond the illusion that traps your soul.

You are reading this book because you are seeking Truth. Not only do you want to know about it, you want to experience it yourself. Everything is a belief until you experience it or understand more deeply. According to Acharya Shree Yogeesh, "All beliefs are false." It's a strong statement. Don't expect anything less than strong in this book. When you know through your soul, with absolute certainty, all doubts, questions and curiosities will leave you. In soul knowing, you are free.

I have been studying under the guidance of Acharya Shree Yogeesh for 10 years now. I have been a monk for almost six years. Through his wisdom, teachings and personal guidance, I not only have changed so much for the better, but I have deeply understood what spirituality is truly about. When I first met him, I loved that he was not a traditional teacher. During our first meeting I asked him if he belonged to any religion. He said, "I am spiritual, not religious." He was the spiritual guide I was seeking. I was raised Catholic, but it didn't answer all of my questions. I despised the politics, the abuse, the control, and greed for money and power. I disapproved of large organizations. To me, I didn't care that many people did not know of him at that time. As long as he could guide me to Truth, to myself, that is all that mattered. Crowds don't give credibility to anyone, anyway. As you will learn in this book, all the crowds flock to misleading teachers. This is not new. Enlightened masters of the past had even warned about this.

Being on the spiritual path is like putting yourself into a burning house to find something that is most precious to you. You will do whatever it takes to find it, even if everything you've loved, learned, or earned burns all around you. It can be painful. But you know that as long as you have this one thing, nothing else matters. That one thing, for me, is soul. I've lost people, I've let go of my ideologies and beliefs that I was raised with for years, I've had to face the darkest parts of me, but I gain myself. Not easy, but worth it. Truth is hard to swallow, but if it's Truth, I'll do whatever it takes to get it. It takes courage. I know you have the courage within you, too.

This book *Chakra Awakening: The Lost Techniques* was initially developed as a supplement to our 14-CD course called *Awaken Chakras* (www.awakenchakras.com). Acharya Shree had asked me, as well as the monks-in-training that live here at Siddhayatan, what we all wanted to know about the chakras. Our Chakra Activation workshop is among the top courses guests come to our retreat for; however, in 3 days not everything could be taught, just the basics. When we initially developed the *Awaken Chakras* audio course, I gave Acharya Shree a list of

2

questions and topics to consider, as he talked more in-depth about the chakras – the typical topics such as what the chakras are, the benefits of knowing about them, and the techniques to balance them. I didn't want him to stop there. I also asked him if he would reveal secrets, hidden teachings, and Truth about the chakras that no one in our modern times knew. With so much junky information out there on the chakras, it is time for the true teachings to be revealed. Spirituality is spirituality. It has everything to do with soul and nothing to do with New Age entertainment.

As I began to edit his audio recordings that contained nearly 12 hours of teachings on the chakras, I noticed my jaw was dropping to the floor all the time. No exaggeration. I would think to myself, "Wait a minute... I never knew that, or that, or that!" I would make sounds like, "Whaat!" "Wow!" "Are you serious?" I was shocked that the world was missing out on so much. The world is trapped. I remember, when I was listening to Acharya Shree's recording when he was specifically revealing the secrets of the chakras, I ran over to him and said, "Are you serious?! I never knew any of this. Why didn't you ever share these teachings? This is huge! It shakes up everything we know about spirituality!" He replied simply and humbly, "You never asked."

True enlightened masters don't just talk or preach to hear themselves speak. They answer the questions of students. Unless a student asks a question, they won't answer. The master also knows if the student is asking out of curiosity and entertainment. In such cases, they may not answer because it would be a waste. When the master sees the student's heart and the sincerity of the question, then he or she will answer. I didn't ask much about the chakras before, because I was personally interested in other aspects of spirituality, like the laws of karma and learning about the higher states of consciousness.

After launching the *Awaken Chakras* course, all of us at Siddhayatan had more questions to what he had given in the audio course. We thought it would be a good idea, then, to publish a book that contained answers to our additional questions that we had after listening to the *Awaken Chakras* audio recordings. We wanted to know the Truth about many more topics, not just the chakras, and we knew many seekers wanted to know the Truth. And now you have that book in your hands.

This book is very important because what you know as spirituality now, may not be the real spirituality. Especially if you have been turning to other sources and teachers for guidance. In this book you will learn about the true origins of spirituality and how they got corrupted and lost over time. You will know the Truth and origins of yoga, the chakra system and the Samanic tradition (monks and nuns who carried spiritual teachings to help awaken the soul).

You will not find these teachings elsewhere because they have been lost and misinterpreted over thousands and thousands of years. Those who teach now are not enlightened so they cannot tell you the history, purpose and safe techniques, and there are only few enlightened masters living at this time (of which none speak English and mostly live in silence, with the exception of Acharya Shree Yogeesh). This statement alone is controversial in itself, because the world continues to be influenced by people who claim to be masters and teachers. There is more damage done than good, especially now, since yoga has become a booming multi-million dollar, if not more, industry.

Acharya Shree Yogeesh has meditated on these Truths and has revived them for you. Through his discourses and discussions on the chakras, his teachings have been compiled by his disciples into this groundbreaking book.

As I said before, it takes courage to know the Truth. Some of it you may disagree with, and that is okay. You are supposed to think. You are

4

supposed to question. When you go whole-heartedly into questioning deeply, that is when you realize the Truth.

You have picked up this book to mostly learn about the chakras. Not only will you get the secrets, hidden teachings and techniques, you will get so many more treasures and gems. It is difficult to put into words how much you will get out of it. I'll just say that this book can be a catalyst for a major turning point in your spiritual path. That in itself changes everything for you.

As you read through *Chakra Awakening: The Lost Techniques*, take notes and read the book over and over again, because you will gain something new each time. Practice what you are learning. You can also go to http://chakraawakeningbook.com/suite to view the activation techniques demonstrated. The way to advance on your path is by practice, not just reading. Practice, not just believing. Practice leads to soul knowing. Soul knowing leads you to Truth.

Awaken your chakras. Awaken yourself.

Sadhvi Siddhali Shree
Chief Disciple of Acharya Shree Yogeesh
Spiritual Director of Siddhayatan Tirth & Spiritual Retreat
Author, 31 Days to a Changed You

INTRODUCTION

The chakra system comes from an ancient tradition of universal spiritual teachings in India. It's a system that has been shared for thousands of years by yogis and monks, but nowadays has been mostly forgotten. When you know how to balance your chakras and fill them with energy you can become healthier – and remember, a healthy body and mind can lead a person towards becoming very spiritual. If you want to put meaning into your life and feel peaceful, it's important to understand the chakra system, which can transform your life and bring you aliveness. When you have aliveness, life becomes moment to moment, and that life is beautiful.

Life is the most precious thing and we need to respect it – especially human life, because it's very difficult to get. You need to understand this. Someone once asked me, "If human life is so difficult to get, then why are there more than six billion people on Earth?" A population like this has never happened before. This is the best time to live, because technology makes it easier to learn and communicate. Many people believe that this is the worst period to be alive, the period of Kali Yuga as it's known in India, but this is incorrect. The reason there is a big population on Earth is because there are many souls that are improving and getting the human body. It's the era of technology and the best time to be spiritual.

In order to grow spiritually and be physically and mentally healthy you need to know about chakras. You can clear your mind of confusion and doubts, have pure thoughts and take yourself higher.

Maybe you're unaware of how many sicknesses and diseases you're carrying, or perhaps you think your body is the healthiest already. Let me tell you that toxins are of many different kinds, and they go into the deepest parts of us and hide, even for many lifetimes, before they start to come on the surface and begin their chaos. You can burn and release these toxins using the universal spiritual teachings you'll find here and then you will have the best body: the body that is clean and strong enough to begin your spiritual path.

Chakras have the potential to help more than any medicine. Medicines will store unwanted things in your body and give you side effects, leaving the cause for your disease untouched or create a further complication in your system. You need your system to be fully clear, otherwise you cannot perceive the truth in what you see and your soul will never get the right message from your senses. You will understand more as you read about this system and where it comes from.

PART I:
THE ORIGINS

PART I:
THE ORIGINS

TIRTHANKARAS

There are many things to understand in the chakra system. Today, chakras are becoming widely popular among yoga practitioners and others who want to live spiritually, but no one understands where the system comes from and it needs to be known. It's a beautiful tradition. Even the kings bowed down in respect to these long-ago monks who worked only to awaken their souls. They embodied the purest virtues, such as nonviolence, forgiveness, truthfulness and compassion, and dedicated their lives to the earnest search of truth in the universe. The path they walked is the most difficult path, taking complete responsibility for their lives and living according to the highest spiritual principles in order to dissolve their karma and reach enlightenment, liberating themselves from the cycle of ignorance, pain, suffering, birth and death.

These were the *Tirthankaras*, *Arihantas* and the monks and nuns, known as *Samanas*, and later *Shramanas* (coming from the Prakrit root for "effort towards the soul"). They sought shelter in the spiritual path after renouncing the world to answer the call of their souls.

Tirthankaras are little known outside of India today, though their teachings have unknowingly affected millions of people throughout the world. Tirthankara is a Sanskrit word meaning "one who makes the harbor." Why make a harbor? If you want to cross the ocean you need to get on a ship, and to get on the ship you must find the harbor. Around the Tirthankara, the *Tirtha* is formed. Tirtha is the harbor, the home of the ship. So the figurative meaning is the ocean of suffering, ocean of pain, and we need to cross it. If we have the right teachings then the crossing becomes possible, otherwise we'll wander here and there, maybe going in the wrong direction. You can also say God; without God you cannot go further, and a Tirthankara is like a living God. You can ask them questions and they will give you guidance for your path and help you to raise your consciousness to the highest state. Without a body, God cannot communicate. Tirthankaras and Arihantas are in that highest state of consciousness because of all the efforts they put to reach enlightenment, but they have the instrument of mind, senses and body – their last body – otherwise it is not possible to communicate with God. People who claim they talk with God, or they hear God's voice and receive messages, they have no idea what the real meaning of God is. God doesn't have a voice. They mislead many people and those people are easily trapped into it because they don't understand what God is either. Instead of raising their consciousness through spiritual practices to become like that, they are just deluding themselves further; they're going in the opposite direction of God.

In our time cycle there were 24 Tirthankaras; the first was *Adinath* and the last was *Vardhaman*, known in Jainism as *Rishabhdeva* and *Mahavira*, respectively. Tirthankaras are born as humans but their bodies are unique. It's the hardest thing in the world to be a Tirthankara. They must go through incredible suffering which is why they have such a unique body; it's very strong and has a structure that is different from ours. It can tolerate so much. They remain balanced and unaffected throughout their suffering, though, because they know that whatever is happening to them is just the result of their karma; they brought it on themselves from their past lives.

Whatever happens to a Tirthankara's body while they're alive will not kill them. This is why I say that Tirthankaras are extraordinary – a kind of "super-human." Until their *ayu karma* dissolves, nothing will kill their bodies. Ayu karma is the karma that determines one's lifespan, but in a normal person's case, they can still die before their ayu karma is finished. The Tirthankara cannot. Their bodies are so strong that even if someone with a modern gun attacked them, the bullets would not penetrate their skin.

Mahavira is a true example to all people on the spiritual path. For all the karma that he had accumulated, reciting mantras was not enough to dissolve it. He had to suffer, and he had to be tortured. He had to go through extreme pain. There is a story from his life, a true story. There was an angel named *Sangam*. In their previous lives together, Mahavira was a king and Sangam was his slave. Even though Sangam was now an angel, he didn't forget how badly he was treated by him. He had so much hate, so much anger, and a thirst for revenge. He wanted to get Mahavira back, and he tried. He tried everything. One day, Mahavira was standing in very deep meditation and Sangam found him. As an angel he was able to transform his body into different shapes, animal bodies, and could even change the nature around. He started bothering Mahavira, but not only bothering him, torturing him. He was willing to do whatever it took to stop Mahavira from meditation. Sangam would bite Mahavira; he changed his shape into a scorpion or a snake. He would change the weather to create huge hailstorms, and all of that hail would pound on Mahavira's body as e was meditating. Sangam even lit the entire forest on fire in order to scare Mahavira and in hopes of burning him. He threw Mahavira up in the air, but when he landed it was the pain of thousands of thorns on his body. Never wasting a single minute, Sangam tried day and night. Not just one day, two days, three days or a week. Not just one week, or two weeks, or one month. He tried for six entire months – every single minute full of torture. Can you imagine Mahavira, for every minute of six months, trying to go deep into meditation and connect with his soul through all of that suffering? And yet he didn't move. All the physical abuse, emotional abuse, mental abuse – Sangam tried everything. We need to learn from Mahavira. He was strong. He didn't even move an inch. It had the opposite effect; with every type of torture, every attack and every bit of excruciating pain, he became stronger and stronger in himself. He began to embody all of his highest qualities. And after six months, Sangam finally gave up. He realized he could not break down Mahavira. He approached him and told him, "I'm leaving now."

Mahavira, standing in deep meditation, slowly opened his eyes and gently looked at Sangam. He said, "You're leaving?"

And to Sangam's surprise, he noticed a tear in Mahavira's eye.

"You never flinched, you didn't make a sound, you didn't even move an inch, and you never retaliated or got angry. I bothered you. I tortured you so much. You're supposed to be happy that I'm leaving. Why are you crying?"

Mahavira replied, "These tears are not because I'm sad that you're leaving. These tears don't come from all the pain you've caused for those entire six months. These tears come, because I see your future lives, and you will suffer so much. You will go through so much pain and torture; – the worst of all the hell-like planets. I'm not crying for myself. I'm crying for you."

Mahavira's words hit Sangam. Mahavira never cried for himself. We can learn from Mahavira that we need to be strong; that no matter what we go through in life, we need to be unshakable.

Although the Tirthankaras are found within Jainism, not one Tirthankara is a religious figure and Jains need to wake up to this. They think that they belong to Jainism and teach the Jain principles to reestablish the religion throughout time. Tirthankaras belong to no one. Maybe the Jains have all blocked their *Sahasrara* chakras and can't let go of that idea to see the reality. It's true that the principles of Jainism are solely spiritual principles that can lead you to *moksha*, or liberation, if you have the right understanding of them, but Tirthankaras never taught anything to do with religion. A Tirthankara only teaches according to the needs of the society in the time period that they live, and they share only spiritual vision to help the individuals grow. They teach universal spiritual teachings which belong to no belief system; anyone can live by these principles and they will see their lives blossom right away.

Usually they are born in a royal family. This is because in order to become a Tirthankara, that soul needs an abundance of virtues, collected over many lifetimes by doing the best things possible, putting their whole heart in it and enjoying it selflessly, as well as doing a lot of work to improve themselves. This is how virtues are collected. Because of these virtues, they have collected a lot of good karma, and as a result they are born into a high family during their time period.

When someone is on the spiritual path, dedicating every moment to improving themselves and indulging whole-heartedly in their *sadhana*, or spiritual practices, they begin to deepen their understanding and catch glimpses of the truth. Slowly, as that person improves they begin to close the sources where karmas flow in to cover their soul. The influence from their senses and mind diminishes and the soul begins to gain strength. Because of the intense sadhana that the soul of a Tirthankara has gone through in its previous lives, when they are born as a Tirthankara, they

15

have three types of knowledge already: *mati jnana, shruti jnana*, and *avadhi jnana*.

Mati jnana means to receive the perfect knowledge that is transmitted through the organs and senses, including the intellect. For example, when you see something, you see it for what it really is. When you hear something, you hear it as it should be heard. It is perfect, crystal-clear perception without any distortion or misunderstanding. A Tirthankara perceives everything 100% perfectly through their organs and senses (eyesight, hearing, smell, taste, and touch); they don't need to think about it or ask any questions. When they have shruti jnana they have the correct perception and interpretation of what is heard. As they learn, they learn correctly and perfectly. Avadhi jnana is the ability to see anything perfectly, up to a certain distance. Maybe it's 1,000 miles away, across the whole Earth or on other planets. It depends on the karma, but it can differ, so it's still considered a limited knowing, not full yet.

Anyone can achieve these if they put the effort to work on themselves, by first cleaning their bodies and then balancing their energy through spiritual practices. The human body is the best instrument to realize enlightenment, but it needs to be very healthy. Soul has unlimited knowing and power. It's never-ending. Unfortunately we have millions of layers of karma that surround our souls and keep them in the dark, but anybody can uncover that power if they have the right guidance and a craving to find the truth. You cannot waste any time. You have to remember that nothing is impossible.

It is in your reach to become an Arihanta, an enlightened person. This word, Arihanta, has a beautiful meaning. Like Tirthankara, Arihanta is also a word coming from the Sanskrit language. "Ari" means "enemies," and "hanta" means "who has destroyed." If you can destroy all of your enemies, then you will reach enlightenment, but how do you know what the real enemy is? A spiritual person knows that their enemies live on the inside. All the inner-phenomena that cause us to suffer, that cause us to doubt ourselves and bring grief upon ourselves or think, speak and act negatively on others, these are the real enemies – anger, greed, ego and jealousy. When we overcome these *kshayas*, the passions that cloud our intentions, then our souls light up. The one who has dissolved all the inner-enemies – that is an Arihanta, or *Arhat*.

A Tirthankara is also an Arihanta, because they have dissolved all of these lower qualities, burned their major karma and reached the highest state of consciousness, but an Arihanta is not necessarily a Tirthankara. Tirthankaras are very rare in the universe. Anyone can become an Arihanta, there is no limit, but at any given time there can only be one Tirthankara on a planet. It's not required that a Tirthankara needs to be present for someone to become enlightened. That person who wants to be on the path simply needs the right guidance. An Arihanta and Tirthankara have the same knowing, they are both in the highest state of consciousness and living in their last bodies, and that is who you need to seek in order to get the right guidance. On our planet there are no Tirthankaras because they cannot be born in this period of time, but there are enlightened masters. I've mentioned before that you can count them on one hand. If you want guidance to take yourself higher, then make an effort to meet a master, an Arihanta.

Mahavira, the 24th and last Tirthankara who was living over 2,600 years ago, initiated many monks that later became enlightened, but told his chief disciple, *Gautam*, that he wouldn't reach enlightenment until he died because he was too attached to him as his teacher. On the day Mahavira left his body and became *Siddha*, a liberated soul, Gautam wept and felt so sad that his teacher was gone. He was thinking, "How are the other monks enlightened and I'm still not? I've been sharing his teachings everywhere and bringing many people to meet him." In his sadness and frustration, he realized his attachment to Mahavira and remembered what he was told. In that moment his attachment dissolved and he became enlightened. All over the world now, this day is celebrated as *Diwali* – the day that Mahavira became liberated, and the day that Gautam reached enlightenment.

Our planet is very lucky. Let me tell you that in the whole universe there can only be a maximum of 170 Tirthankaras. Not just in our solar system, but the whole universe. There are millions and millions of galaxies in the universe if you could only see them. Out of these, some can tolerate more than others – it depends. Many planets cannot tolerate the energy of having a Tirthankara living there because it's too much. Some planets are able to tolerate a Tirthankara always; as soon as the last Tirthankara becomes Siddha (leaves their body and merges with all the other liberated souls), the next one is born. Unlike the other planets that have long gaps of time in between each Tirthankara, there are no gaps in between on these 20 planets. So, a minimum of 20 Tirthankaras will remain in the universe at all times, because of these unique planets. This is why there is a maximum and minimum number of Tirthankaras in the universe at any time; 20 planets have a Tirthankara at all times, and just 170 planets can even tolerate the energy.

Tirthankaras will never meet each other, because there can only be one living on a planet at a time, but they can communicate easily. An enlightened master has that ability. Consider how fortunate we are that our planet here can tolerate that energy, and on top of that we've had 24 Tirthankaras on Earth in this period of time alone. Presently there are no Tirthankaras on our planet because they're not born in this era. If someone has the yogic power, though, they can travel in the universe to find them, and in their presence they will really understand what the Tirthankara is;

you dive deep into your consciousness where only stillness, tranquility, calmness and peace prevail. You feel the truth.

Jains are wrong in this case to fix the number that there will be 24 Tirthankaras in each time cycle. It just happened that way in our last time period. It doesn't necessarily mean there will be another 24 again and again. There is no such thing as a set number. Each cycle comes and goes and the history is lost repeatedly; people only think of recent times. What about before then? What if there is just one Tirthankara in the next cycle? It's wrong to say there's a set number. It depends on karma.

I can't show you, but I can tell you, when the Tirthankara is sitting they have something which no other kind of body has. Suppose when someone is sitting in a cross-legged position, like lotus posture, with both hands in their lap, their shoulders broadly open and their arms relaxed on their sides, their knees will be wider than the rest of their body and their elbows won't touch to their knees. But this isn't the way a Tirthankara's body is. Everywhere is an equal distance; from shoulder to shoulder, down to one knee and across to there other knee is like a square. Normally people who are born on Earth don't have a body like that. It only happens with a Tirthankara. The statues that I see are not made the right way, because if you were to measure shoulder to shoulder, arms to knees, and knee to knee while sitting in lotus posture, it would be all equal measurements. In India it's not their fault the statues are done incorrectly because nobody knows the truth. They aren't knowledgeable about Tirthankaras – not the real things.

They're born as a human but with the extraordinary body. As soon as it's time for them to renounce their life in royalty and continue their sadhana again, they leave the kingdom and simply recite, *"Siddhanam Namo Kiccha."* They don't need to be initiated onto the spiritual path by anybody. They do it for themselves. Upon their renunciation they achieve the fourth type of knowing, *manas paryaya jnana*; they see all the particles of the mind, even if a person is very far away. All the particles are seen clearly, all the thoughts. They're like images, and move through the air like bubbles going here and there. That's why sometimes people can have the same thought at the same moment, like when two close friends think of the same thing. They're catching the thought as it moves. When you have this knowing, manas paryaya jnana, you can see the thought particles everywhere.

One Tirthankara was enlightened in the very moment he renounced the world. Sometimes Tirthankaras have to put a lot of effort in order to achieve their enlightenment. It's not as easy as simply gazing in the mirror and asking questions. For example, the first Tirthankara Adinath went without food or water for one year and then achieved his enlightenment. So each Tirthankara has a different life, but it doesn't mean some of them have an easier life. It depends on their karma, and they are balanced anyway. Whatever happens, if people are praising them and bowing, or even torturing them, they remain balanced and unaffected. To get the life of a Tirthankara you have to put a lot of effort on the spiritual path and collect the best karma. Don't be confused about it; your goal is supposed to be the highest state of consciousness, it is just an example to show you how much those souls go through. Whether you become a Tirthankara or you reach enlightenment as an every-day person, it makes no difference. Enlightenment is enlightenment. Bliss is bliss. In Mahavira's case it took him 27 lifetimes once he began his path, and then 12-and-a-half years of intense sadhana as a Tirthankara before he reached enlightenment, but he remained balanced always. That is how you dissolve karma. You have to be completely balanced and equal, even if a good thing is happening or a bad thing. You don't want to collect good karma or bad karma, because it will continue carrying you from life to life; you want to stop collecting karma completely, and burn whatever remaining karma you have from the past. It's hard to understand what Mahavira had to go through during his years of sadhana. If you combine the karma of all 23 Tirthankaras before him, his was much heavier.

From the moment they renounce to the moment enlightenment is realized, they don't speak at all. They know they don't have perfect knowing and only want to indulge in their sadhana. After that, they might speak only a few words if somebody asks a question, but even by just being in their presence people learn a lot of things. Your soul can be really affected in the presence of an enlightened master, even if you don't know who they are.

When many people come to be around a Tirthankara for *Samvasaran*, it's very special. Samvasaran is a spiritual gathering of all kinds of species. It only happens around a Tirthankara. They all come to be in a huge circle around the Tirthankara and they learn from their presence. Monks and nuns, laypeople, all the different kinds of angels, animals and even bugs who are present; everyone is in calmness and peace. In the presence of a Tirthankara, the ego is forgotten, animosity disappears, everything is dropped and everyone is equal. A mongoose and a snake, born enemies, will forget about it. The lion will lose its desire to kill the goat. This only happens with a Tirthankara and no one else. It's a kind of miracle that happens around them.

There are 34 different *atishaya* that happen around a Tirthankara; atishaya means a kind of miraculous happening. Tirthankaras don't create these miracles, they just happen. Nobody can create miracles. Whoever claims they can make miracles is already wrong. Miracles can never be created, they can only happen. Remember not to get trapped into listening to someone who is claiming to do miracles. Everything is drawn to the Tirthankara. It's difficult to understand what they really are. If I try to describe them, the best thing to say is, in the whole universe, you find all of the best possible particles, the purest particles, and bring all of them into just one body. You cannot imagine how extraordinary a Tirthankara is. If they go to sit on the ground somewhere, the ground always comes up to support them. They go to walk, but some flowers or grass always grows under their feet. Wherever they pass, even dead things that never blossom will begin to blossom again. Some diseases will disappear from the region where they are, and wars between kingdoms will stop. There are many things, and it is hard to believe, but they actually happen.

There are many planets, we call them heavenly planets, where there is no suffering at all, only pleasure, and the pleasure you find on our planet is nothing in comparison to that kind of place. These are the planets where angels are born. When you are born as an angel, I always call it a vacation; you get a little break from your suffering, but it's a big waste of time for your soul. Sometimes you can be on those planets for millions of years, just in pleasure, because you cannot follow spirituality when you don't experience suffering. Angels cannot follow spirituality. You go on vacation and all these years pass by where you could be doing sadhana instead. You don't want that kind of vacation, you want to be born as a human so you can reach enlightenment. Angels cannot do it, so they are really shocked and impressed when someone is on the path and into it fully. They rarely ever come by our planet, but it happens from time to time. When there is a Tirthankara, they are amazed and they want to serve the Tirthankara. That is how all of these atishaya happen, because when you have an angel body, you can change things around. Another atishaya of the Tirthankara is that when there are many people around and they speak about something, they talk in a way that everybody can understand them. Today we have a special earpiece that immediately translates what you're hearing into your own language. That happens when the

Tirthankara speaks, so everyone can understand. These things only happen around a Tirthankara; all of the angels – they're called *devas* in India – rush to do things for them in every moment. They create the Samvasaran and bring many other angels and animals around, where they create a beautiful place for everyone to absorb the spiritual teachings. Everyone can hear the teachings clearly, no matter if they are sitting in front of the Tirthankara or far away. As soon as the Samvasaran is finished everything goes back to normal.

The particles of their bodies are so light they have only a faint shadow after enlightenment. If it's wintertime when they're walking somewhere then nothing will grow, but if it's the right season then many dead plants, flowers, crops and vegetation will begin to blossom and come to life after being affected by their energy. Wherever the Tirthankara is found, for a certain distance around them there will be the feeling of calmness.

To be a disciple of a Tirthankara feels like you are in a kind of light always; you have the benefit to live with an extraordinary person on the Earth and learn directly from their presence. Their entire life is spent in sadhana, discipline, meditation and working to dissolve their karma. It is the most difficult thing in the universe to be on the spiritual path and discover the soul that is sleeping inside you. Nothing can be compared to a Tirthankara, because their bodies are totally different to endure a lot of things. When you're with them you feel as if you're in the presence of the living-God and you get that kind of inspiration always. Tirthankaras are not born on our planet in this time, but if you put enough effort to find the enlightened master who can guide you, then you will go through the same process as if you were with one of them. Because an Arihanta and Tirthankara are both enlightened, there is no difference in their knowing; they both are seated in the highest state of consciousness, so you will learn the same things that you need in order for your soul to gain strength and blossom. It is a difficult process, and it's very hard to live with a master, because they will react. Whatever mistakes you're doing, they will make you aware of it. Most people just surrender to God, but their God is just a thing someplace else; it doesn't react to them, so it's very easy to surrender to that God.

To reach enlightenment, the enlightened person will make you shake inside, so you begin to see that reality is not what you think. It's not by reading the Gita, or the Bible, or just having devotion merely. That is not enough. You have to go through the process with a lot of effort and determination. No one has ever reached enlightenment through scriptures and rituals alone. Those are just wastage of time. A Tirthankara and their monks and nuns don't perform any kind of rituals, and what is the point to wasting your time repeating scriptures to try and understand the meaning when you can get the real truth directly from your teacher? They will say it in the way that will make you get the meaning, too, because they know what words will affect you. These things, rituals and scriptures, don't take you anywhere, but unfortunately people get stuck in them easily. Nowadays people see someone who knows the Sanskrit language and is a scholar of the Gita, and they consider them to be enlightened. These people don't even know what enlightenment is. The real enlightenment, when your soul gains all its strength, is hard to understand. You need to have the right concept of it or else you will do things that lead you elsewhere. With a Tirthankara, after a while, if someone is wise enough they may compile some of their teachings by memorizing and passing them along. If monks or nuns throughout time did so, most of the teachings have been lost.

It's unfortunate that their teachings were lost, but it's not up to them. They lived in that time and they taught in that time. After that, whatever the situation is throughout history, droughts or disasters or other things, the teachings get lost through it all. People die in the disasters or from diseases that spread across the lands. If there were monks and nuns who were carrying the real teachings after the Tirthankara's body died, they go through a lot of things, too. Maybe no one ever asked those monks and nuns any good questions, or maybe they didn't really come across other people often. So, things like this happen and they eventually die, too, and the teachings with them. Whatever is left over eventually trickles together through many different people but becomes confusing because they have interpreted it in the wrong way.

Spiritual teachings are not confusing. The principles of someone who is on the spiritual path are not confusing, but when people ask questions about the universe, other planets, emotions, the mind, this and that, then it can become confusing, because everyone's mind works in a different way. Tirthankaras will answer only if someone asks a question, but most often when people are in their presence, they feel so much peace that they forget their questions. From time to time someone will ask something and if anybody else is there then they'll hear, too, but maybe they interpret it wrongly because it wasn't their own question. Many things are misinterpreted and become confusing later when scriptures are compiled. The teachings that are available in Jain scriptures in the present time are teachings from Mahavira mostly. All the teachings from the other Tirthankaras are not remembered because much time has passed since they were here. If we had a lot of teachings in detail from the other Tirthankaras they could be totally different. It depends on their time period and what the people were like then. The principles will never change, but the way they taught them will.

Mahavira was living in such a harsh way and told his monks not to imitate him, because he was doing what only his body could tolerate, and for the specific karmas he had left to dissolve. But living with the

Tirthankara and following their example is the only way monks and nuns learn from them; they sit in meditation and don't go for food, so the monks and nuns will do the same. They didn't think about fasting, they just copied the Tirthankara. If they didn't go for food, then they wouldn't either. They learned a lot of tolerance and discipline this way. Mahavira had a lot of karma to go through, so he had to be extreme in his sadhana. Other people copied what he was doing and all of the Jain scriptures today reflect Mahavira's teachings in this way. One Tirthankara's teachings will never contradict another Tirthankara's teachings, but they may be totally different because of the needs of the people and the way they had to live to burn their own karmas. Jains got too stuck into *kriyas*, actions. They don't walk here, or they don't touch this dirt or touch this water. Today if a householder gives them alms to eat, and they touch the fire from cooking by accident, the monk will refuse to eat the food, because it goes against their rules of begging food. Those monks are so blind they don't even see how much suffering they cause the householder, because the whole day they will feel bad about their mistake if the monk refuses their food. It is part of the 42 rules for a monk to follow when collecting alms, all coming from Mahavira's time, what he had to go through. And the householders are even more blind because of the monks refusal to accept their food. They begin to think they are the best monks in the universe, because they're so strict. These things mesmerize people in India. It is all just show. It doesn't mean anything. It's unfortunate that the Tirthankaras' teachings become distorted in this way, but it is not up to them. People need to wake up and see what they are doing. Remember, merely kriyas without understanding is blind. That is what Mahavira said, "Padhaman nanam tao daya." This means, "First understand. Then do the kriyas. Then follow futile rules."

A Tirthankara and Arihanta share spiritual principles that can be

practiced by every single person on the planet. They are not based in beliefs or ideas or theories. Rather, they are slow steps to lead you out of your box that you have spent so much time building around your soul – all of the darkness, the ignorance, all of the karma. These spiritual principles are the basic teachings that will help you to stop collecting karma if you practice them with your whole heart. Every moment we collect karma – through our thoughts, our emotions, the words we speak and the actions we do. All of these combined with our constantly-wavering intentions attract millions of karmic particles that cover our soul. You need the purest intention always if you want to raise your consciousness to the highest state and break the karma that keeps you from being free. There is not one moment in life where we are not collecting karma, unless somehow you are able to go deep into meditation. The spiritual principles you can learn from the Tirthankaras and other enlightened people will lift you to that highest state, where like the clouds you will dissolve yourself. If you are fortunate enough to learn from these extraordinary people in your life, you should be very grateful that you are blessed. It is not easy to get a human life, and on top of that it is even more difficult to listen to the truth. Our souls go through many things which we don't understand or even realize, but if we can take the teachings of the Tirthankaras and dive into them with our whole being to understand and practice them, one day we will see with crystal-clear vision and experience the truth like the brave ones who have responded to the call of their soul through time before us.

TIRTHANKARA SHRI ADINATH AND THE BEGINNING

There are countless paths to enlightenment – as many as there are souls. If you hold out your hand and think about the space of air just above your palm, there are infinite souls in that small space. And if you hold out your other hand and see the same space of air, there are infinite souls there also. Just like this, the different paths to moksha, or liberation, are many. It is difficult to understand soul; it is light, but it has no source of light. If you light a candle or a matchstick, or turn a light on, you can see from where the light comes. The soul is different from this. It has no source and no origin.

Even though each person experiences spirituality differently, everyone has talked about his or her soul in some way. We say that things touch our soul deeply. It means we are hit by something and feel it reaching into our depths. If you're fortunate, maybe something in your life will catch you so strongly and take you inward and shake your being. You might begin to see the world around you in a new perspective. Maybe your heart will even begin to blossom and perhaps you'll take responsibility for all of your thoughts, words and actions and choose to live spiritually. This is the hardest thing, but it can be done. Every path is different; everyone has to go through different things. Inside each person is a completely different universe of thoughts, emotions and experiences. We all have different bodies and different minds, so you have to find the right guidance in order to complete the journey; you need to find the harbor where you can go board your ship.

India is known for its spiritual culture. Many saints and yoga masters come from this culture, and in the West, especially, people who don't know any better praise them as gods. Over the last century, some of them have come to the United States, Europe and many other countries to spread their messages. Even though they all come from India, their teachings seem to contradict each other, and even fewer of these teachers follow their own teachings. Many get their teachings from Sikh or Hindu texts, some praise Patañjali and recite the Yoga Sutras to their students, while others attract many followers by inspiring them with make-believe spiritual heroes from the peaks of the Himalayan mountains and tell stories of their feats. Many Westerners simply find an Indian scholar of the Gita and accept them as their guru. They are just reciting lines out of a book, but to a foreign person they can't tell the difference. Whoever has the heart of the truth-seeker might have a chance to get past all of these trappings if they're wise enough, but many don't. If you don't know the history of where these systems and teachings come from, then you will be easily stuck on your path.

The many beliefs that come from India can be confusing to many truth-seekers, though somehow they know that India is where spirituality has blossomed in the past. Many travel there seeking a *guru*, or spiritual teacher, to guide them through their experiences and take them to enlightenment, but how will the seeker realize truths if their heads are being filled with the wrong concepts and false teachings? They are filling up their minds when they should be emptying them. They talk about Shiva, Krishna and Ganesha, yet they don't know who they really were; they only know myths that were created about them. Hindus and Jains are ignorant of the truth, too. If you really want to be on the spiritual path and awaken your soul, then you need to have the right concept in your mind before you can go beyond it. If you want to be healthy and clean and make your body fit to experience higher states of consciousness, then you need to know the origins of the chakra system to understand where these teachings are coming from and how they will benefit you. Don't be trapped. Is it coming from Hinduism? Hindu is a very new word. Who were the real teachers? I can tell you that the truth about it is far from what you have heard. These things have been forgotten.

History as the world knows it is very limited; five thousand or ten thousand years is not a long time. These are the only recorded things that are available to us. This planet is constantly changing, and throughout time there are many societies and civilizations that are not remembered because the circumstances have taken all of the records. Civilizations come and go, it is nothing new. Suppose you're driving home from work and there's a car accident on the road. Who will know what really happened? The police will interview someone there and ask them what happened, and that person will tell them it was a hit-and-run, and the car was blue, or maybe red. Another person will say it was the other driver's fault. The police have to ask everybody there what happened, and you'll end up with fifty people who all give a different story. And that is happening today. You think that people will know what happened one or two thousand years ago? It's not even very far from our time. So history is like that. I always suggest to people to try and get the right understanding of things. We don't need the history books that are read today. Just go deep within yourself and you will gain the vision to see how things really happen.

There was a time on this Earth where spirituality did not exist. No one thought about the soul, or what God is. Those ideas were not here. First, you have to understand that millions of years ago in the time when the first Tirthankara, Adinath, was born, there was no society. People used to live in many different tribes. They lived only to continue surviving; there was no system of living or being civilized – just to hunt and find shelter. The leaders of the tribes were called *Kulkar*. It means head of the tribe, or clan. In that time there were fourteen main Kulkar. Nabhiraja was the name of the last Kulkar, before his son Adinath.

In the tribes they lived like cave people and were not civilized at all. Adinath did something that had never happened on Earth before. He brought all of the tribes together as one, becoming the leader of all the people, and thus beginning the first era of society.

Actually, Adinath is the same person as who Hindus call Shiva, but their idea is totally wrong. "Adi" means "first": the first one to start the era, to bring the civilization together. He brought them from their ignorance and harsh way of living into a beautiful society full of vision, understanding and compassion. In Christianity they think of Adam, the first human. See how it happens? Adi and Adam have the same root. In Arabic it becomes Aadam, or also Adem, the first prophet or first person in civilization. Adinath means "First Lord." Every major religion carries this name, because he was the first to start civilization on Earth. Everything started with him and his name was remembered in all the traditions.

In order to bring the tribes together he taught them three things: *asi,* *masi* and *krisi*. These were the three systems needed in order to create the civilization and flourish. Adinath taught them asi – to protect themselves and their families with whatever they had available to use. Maybe it was

32

just carved stones or long pointed spears. If they didn't have the idea to protect their lives, then they would not last long as a group. Masi means ink – to make drawings or designs, and krisi is agriculture. Before this, no one farmed or knew how to grow things and use the land and climate to their advantage. People didn't have the luxury to think about these things because they were busy surviving. This is the beginning of the first civilization in our time cycle.

The people then were so innocent like children. They didn't know much or understand things, so they had to be taught again and again, not to do this, not to do that. A child will understand one thing, but not another thing. Most of the time they did not understand him as their leader, but they respected him so much and were eager to learn from him.

There is a story of two monks who were innocent like this. Monks used to collect alms once a day. That was the only time they ate, and some still practice this today. They would start walking to wherever they could go, sometimes early in the morning, and by the time they arrived in a town, the people would be eating their lunch and would have food available to give to monks. They would have to walk miles and miles for their meal sometimes. Two monks were once told by their teacher not to come back late in the dark after collecting alms. On their way back, they saw an acrobat performer dancing on a rope and couldn't stop watching. That night their teacher scolded them for being late and asked what happened. They answered honestly about watching the person dancing and mentioned that they didn't realize much time had passed until it was dark already. Their teacher told them not to watch those kinds of things, because it distracts them from completing their responsibilities. The monks apologized so much, they felt very bad. They said they understood and it wouldn't happen again. The next day the very same thing happened. Coming back at night they were late by two hours, and upon being seen, their teacher asked them again why they were late. They replied that on the way they saw a female acrobat dancing on a rope and it was so beautiful and amazing that they couldn't stop watching. The teacher became very furious.

"I told you not to watch it!" he scolded them.

"But you said not to watch the male dancer; you didn't mention about the female dancer!"

They didn't get that it meant both things. Again, they apologized and felt sorry. That's what the people were like with Adinath – very innocent. When people are innocent like this they can be very spiritual if they have guidance. Whatever Adinath was teaching them, they accepted it. No one resisted him at all because they respected him too much and wanted to learn.

With the introduction of agriculture into their lives, the whole society slowly became vegetarian. Remember that Tirthankaras are born with three types of knowing: mati jnana, shruti jnana and avadhi jnana. When a person goes through a lot of experiences in life and they get hit deeply by something, when they have a realization, they see that all of the things in life that were once normal to them now seem like distractions from the real purpose. They turn inward and begin to do spiritual practices and learn how to dissolve their karma in order to realize soul and become enlightened. In the case of a Tirthankara, they know right away that they will renounce one day because of their knowing. They don't have to realize anything in society to light a spark in them; they do what needs to be done in the meantime and wait for the right moment when they can renounce and pick up their sadhana again. Adinath was teaching the people how to live together in a community and learn new abilities so they could thrive. He was the king and brought a little law. At this time there were still no spiritual teachings, because he hadn't renounced yet. If someone was doing something that was not accepted, people would simply glare their eyes at them and the wrongdoer would stop; they couldn't stand to feel shame or to do something against the other people. Or, they would say, "*dhikka,*" or "*dhikkaar.*" It was considered the harshest punishment. It means the same as when someone says, "shame on you." It was enough, because no one wanted to hear it. Laws were not needed much, but there were a few small things like this. People respected the few laws and felt disrespected in society if they ever heard that word spoken to them.

When the people became organized in this way, from tribes into the society, Adinath began ruling over the civilization as king. Enlightened people have a lot of vision; they can see many things in distant time and understand situations clearly. Before Adinath married there was no family system of husband and wife, brothers, sisters or anything like this. It was just the couple that was born together. Everyone was born as twins then; it was in their genes and had something to do with eating meat. Many animals have more than one baby. Cats can have five or six, and dogs are the same, too. Usually these animals are more meat-eaters. When you slowly go towards vegetarianism, that gene line is broken, and multiple babies won't be born as often, mostly just one. People can still be born as twins nowadays, that's sure, but it's more rare than it used to be. In Adinath's time everyone was born as twins. The twins grew up and became the mother and father, because the idea of brother and sister didn't exist. There was the desire to come together only once in their life. Again twins would be born and they would later become mother and father. Adinath broke this idea. Farming their own food helped to change their diets and people left meat behind fully. Over time these ideas were broken because their bodies and minds became clearer without the toxins that meat carries. When Adinath married, the family system was introduced and slowly, people understood they couldn't be with their twin.

Two daughters and two sons were born to Adinath: Brahmi, Sundari, Bharata and Gommatesha. Once society was at the right place, he renounced the kingdom and gave it to Gommatesha, who followed him and renounced soon after, leaving the kingdom in the hands of his brother, Bharata. From Bharata comes *Bhaarat* – "shining one." This is the other official name of India today.

Through his teachings of asi, masi and krisi, the society was eventually put together and the time came for Adinath to renounce and continue his sadhana. When he left the kingdom many other princes renounced also and became monks. They followed Adinath wherever he went. He recited, "Siddhanam Namo Kiccha," and initiated himself onto the spiritual path. Once a Tirthankara renounces, they won't speak again until they're enlightened. They know they have not realized their soul yet and still have many karmas left to burn. People have a misunderstanding today of enlightened people. It is not necessary that someone becomes enlightened and suddenly attracts many people and begins to teach them. When you really go deep in yourself, you see there is no purpose. The Tirthankaras are putting all of their effort to burn the last of their karma, and after that they will only speak if someone is asking a question, and they say only what the person needs to hear. So, now with Adinath there are thousands of monks and they are going door to door through the kingdom to collect alms. What do you think they gave him? This was the first civilization so they don't know about monks yet. They knew that this was Adinath, their leader, so the people were giving him jewels and things like this, but he refused it. Nobody ever thought to give him food or water. He was walking day after day, and no one thought about it. All the monks with him started thinking that he doesn't even say anything, or ask for food to eat or for water even, what kind of life is this? They slowly began to leave him because they were scared to starve.

Adinath was sharing the system of sadhana. If you go without food or water, this is *tapa*, fasting. If you confess truly from your heart, meditate and do all these things he was sharing, you can become enlightened and be in the highest state of consciousness. How to remove karmas and awaken the soul, this is what he was sharing. In the beginning they were called *Tapasa*, meaning, "one who is always engaged in austerities," and also *Samana*. Coming from the Prakrit language, Samana means "effort." Who puts all the efforts, and where? This is the *Samanic* system, the spiritual path. You can also call it the *Shramanic* system; later on they were called Shramana, which is from Sanskrit and has the same meaning. This system is for putting all the effort towards awakening the soul. Samanas never lived in society or with other people. They lived outside of the cities, in the forests or mountains, wherever they went. People would come to visit them and learn. In that time period it worked, but to be a monk is different now. The sadhana and spiritual principles don't change, but the way of life changes. There are three traditions left now and they all stem from the Samanic system: Jain, Buddhist, and Saṁkhya. Monks and nuns were known as both Samanas and Tapasas. Shramanas became known as Jains later, and now they're known as *sadhvi* and *sadhu*. Sadhvi is a female, and sadhu is a male. Somehow the word *muni* started later for male Samanas. These things came from the system Adinath first taught. When he left his body, the teachings were practiced and carried on by the Samanas – monks and nuns.

Samanic is the purest system, because the monks and nuns work merely on awakening the soul and burning their karma to reach enlightenment. They realize something deeper about life and they want to end their suffering, so they leave the material kind of life behind for the spiritual path, and accept that they have to take responsibility for the karmas they go through. Since the beginning, the Samanic system has been towards enlightenment only. The *Brahmanic* tradition was there in Adinath's time, too, but even in the beginning they were already focused more on rituals to collect money. Brahmans think by performing rituals they can collect good karma, or wealth or good fortune, but this idea is totally wrong. These days the Brahmans don't even want to perform rituals; they're mostly educated and work in business. They feel that performing rituals degrades them, because they think they're higher than that. Mostly, the priests of the lower Brahman class are doing the rituals. Being a priest just means that you take care of the temple or the church, cleaning, doing ceremonies; they're all rituals and have nothing to do with spirituality. Samanas never lived in society or performed rituals.

Samanas couldn't leave the path and still live with the monk clothes, so the ones who began to leave Adinath started to dye their clothes. They started wearing red and orange from the dyes, whatever natural things they could find. In that time it was a symbol of weakness to wear colors like this. These monks that left knew they were weak because they couldn't tolerate the discipline of following Adinath around. The color is known as *garewa* – the color of swamis' clothing. The first one to leave him was his own grandson, Bharata's son, Maarichi. When he left and colored his clothes, Bharata became outraged when he saw him again. He had left his grandfather's teachings. Maarichi said he would die because he has gone so long without food. Bharata never respected him again after he left.

Maarichi had lived with Adinath for a while in the beginning, and was well known because Bharata was the *chakravarti*, a great ruler or king, so many people started coming to him and asking to be his disciple. He was the first swami. It didn't happen because he wanted to create his own group, it was because he was too weak to face his karma and tolerate hunger and thirst, so he left Tirthankara Shri Adinath. All the monks who left respected Adinath still, but they could not do it. They didn't leave for bad reasons or to teach their own ideas. This is where all the sects started. Everything comes from Adinath's system.

Food and water wasn't given to the monks, because no one realized they might be hungry or thirsty. They gave nice things that were denied because the monks didn't need them. What use does jewelry or gold have to a monk? Adinath one day came to Hastinapura, a town in the area where Delhi is today. Another of his grandsons was a ruler there. When he came to his kingdom, there was so much sugarcane. Even still today there is a lot of sugarcane in that region. His grandson offered him sugarcane juice and since Adinath had been fasting for a year, when he broke it with the juice he got so much energy and shortly after he became enlightened. Before a Tirthankara is enlightened they don't initiate anybody on the spiritual path, but now a lot of people came back to him and he initiated them as his disciples.

Maarichi knew deep down in his heart that his path was not good, because he left the enlightened person and knew he was not doing the right thing. Because he was well known already, people still came to him from everywhere to learn, but he sent them away. In his whole life, Maarichi didn't initiate a single person, but he inspired thousands and thousands to start their path. When they came to him he sent them to Adinath. He would tell them they couldn't learn anything from him, but if they really wanted to become a monk and learn some spiritual teachings then they should go to Adinath. Maarichi knew Adinath was enlightened, and from all the thousands of people he inspired to become monks he collected the best karma. That soul which was Maarichi later became Mahavira, the 24th Tirthankara. He was so into what he was doing; he never wanted people to follow him or be his disciple, he just wanted to tell people to go to the real enlightened person.

One day, Bharata asked Adinath in the Samvasaran, spiritual gathering, "Will anyone out of the thousands of people here ever be enlightened?"

Adinath told him the last person sitting over there, not only will he be enlightened, but he will be a Tirthankara and a chakravarti. He told Bharata that this person he was talking about was his own son, Maarichi. He has the ability but he doesn't know it yet. Bharata went to him and bowed down for the first time to his son. He didn't even say anything first, he just bowed. Maarichi was shocked.

"Don't be egoistic; I'm not bowing to you. In the future you will be a Tirthankara. That is who I am bowing down to."

When Bharata left, his son became so proud and celebrated. He was thinking, "My grandfather is a Tirthankara, my father is a chakravarti, but I will be both!"

After this he collected a lot of bad karma in his life from being too proud and had to go through a lot of things before becoming the 24th Tirthankara, Mahavira.

All the sects throughout time and all traditions started here. Within one year of renouncing his kingdom and continuing his sadhana, everything spread. After Adinath broke his fast and began teaching how to ignite the soul, it all started. Before Adinath there was no such thing as spirituality. He was the very first monk and taught people to do sadhana and wake up their souls.

Jains know Adinath as Rishabhdeva. "Rishabh" means "the bull." This was Adinath's symbol. Why do Tirthankaras have a symbol? Jains are so ignorant in this case; Tirthankaras are not born with a symbol. The symbol represents what kind of people were in the society at the time. In Adinath's time people were like bulls. A bull is considered to be an innocent animal and it will fulfill its duty no matter what happens. Give him food, don't give him food, or even keep from giving him water, it doesn't make a difference because the bull will continue going. This is what the people were like. In those days they carried heavy loads all day and night, and the bull has that kind of loyalty to finish his work. If he's carrying a lot of weight, he will keep on carrying, even if he dies on the way. Horses are not like that. A horse won't go further; if they're thirsty you have to stop to give them water and rest. No wonder the symbol of the bull was given to Adinath. The donkey on the other hand will not fulfill its work. It's a very cunning animal and will find ways around it. So, the bull represents the society. All the people were innocent and child-like. Hindus are ignorant, too, because they carry the same symbol for Shiva. There are many similarities with Adinath and the myths about Shiva; it shows that they are the same person. They gave Shiva's bull a different name: *Nandi.* You can say Rishabhdeva or Nandi. Both mean the bull. Jains know the first Tirthankara as Rishabhdeva, but his actual name was Adinath. Hindus think that Shiva used to ride on a bull and they have many stories about this. If people really wanted to know the truth, they could do it, but no one wants to find it. They want to stay with their own ideas. Shiva also had two sons, Ganesha and Kartikeya. After Adinath renounced, Gommatesha followed his father everywhere. He was always with him learning and doing his spiritual practice. Same thing, in the Hindu myths about Shiva, Ganesha was always with him.

When Hinduism was re-established in the eighth century by Adi Shaṁkaracharya, they became so powerful and rejected all the other books. They tried to put the Jain and Buddhist traditions down. Otherwise how could they become the most popular? They tried to find many excuses to put them down. The Hindus felt disrespected for almost 1,300 years, because the society knew they were not real monks. They were just doing rituals, and the Samanic monks were respected more than the greatest kings, so after many years the Brahmans were tired of it. They became so strong and were putting everyone down. They started saying that Shiva is the real thing; they didn't want to hear Adinath's name anymore. Hinduism didn't want to be connected with Samanas, so they tried to make the name Shiva more popular. First of all, Shiva means, "absolute-consciousness"; it's not even a name. If you become Shiva one day, then you are enlightened. They didn't go away from the real meaning, but they didn't want to accept it then, and still today they don't want to accept that Shiva is Adinath. Hopefully one day they might begin to realize the truth.

Gommatesha was a son of Adinath, and brother of Bharata. He is known as *Bahubali* by Jains, and he renounced the kingdom after ruling for a few years when Adinath first left. It's a long story, but somehow he realized it's not worth the struggle and even his own brother wanted the kingdom from him. He realized it was only greediness, and thought that it's better to just leave it for his brother and renounce. He stood for one year in *kayotsarga* position without moving, determined to reach enlightenment. He knew that the rest of his sisters and cousins were already monks and he didn't want to bow to them. When you become a monk, you bow to all the monks who are senior to you, even if they took initiation just one day before you. Gommatesha had ego about it and he wanted to be the first to be enlightened, so he avoided going to them and stood in kayotsarga for one year. He was thinking that when he is enlightened he won't have to bow to anyone. It was his ego.

One day his sisters Brahmi and Sundari went to ask Adinath if anybody in the area would be enlightened. Adinath told them, "There is one person, but he needs a little help. He's riding on an elephant and won't get enlightened until he comes down."

He told Brahmi and Sundari where this person was, and when they

42

went to see him, they realized it was their own brother Gommatesha. They approached him in his meditation and said that he needed to get off his elephant or he won't be enlightened.

"Hey... I am standing – I'm not riding on an elephant."

Gommatesha didn't get it, but he began to think more deeply. It took him a couple of days to find out what kind of elephant he was riding, and he realized finally that the elephant was his ego. He already renounced all the things in life, left his kingdom and was doing his sadhana. Whom to bow to is ridiculous, so he said forget it. As soon as he decided, he didn't even take one step and he reached enlightenment, because ego was the last block for him.

His true name was Gommatesha, and he stuck around Adinath always. Hindus know him by the name of Ganesha, and another popular name in central India, *Ganapati*. There was a time when Hinduism didn't have a stronghold. Most kings in Mahavira's time were Jains or Buddhists, and these kings ruled over India for about 1,100 to 1,300 years. In those days the Brahmans were at a point of being fully outraged. Since the beginning, they were not respected in the same way as Samanas, because the society knew they didn't have the real teachings that can take a person to liberation from the cycle. The kings were even devotees of the Tirthankaras and monks. So, the Brahmans wanted to get more respect and power, and began to distort history, writing against the Samanas. Brahmanic scholars wanted to re-establish Hinduism, but how? They needed to create a lot of fear. If you look into history you will see there are many stories about scaring people into converting by using fear. They would tell people that their families would die if they didn't worship Shiva or Ganesha, or that they would get a bad disease or lose their money, and other things like this. It happened because in Adinath's time when he renounced and started teaching about sadhana, there were two traditions that began. One was the Samanic system and the other was the Brahmanic tradition. The Brahmans were doing a little sadhana, but were more into doing rituals. They were not real monks. The real monk is fearless. They put all their effort, day after day, to improve themselves and awaken their soul. So the two traditions began. One was the system to work on yourself and awaken your soul, and the other was rituals. Eventually, the Brahmans began to think that they were disrespected by society. They created all the mythology in order to get more respect than the monks. Also, a few bad muslim kings hired Brahmans to write books in order to distort Indian history. All those Brahmans who were greedy for money ruined their own country's history and mythology. Later on, the common Indian people believe these lies to be true. Why does a monk need respect? If they get respect or if they don't get respect, it doesn't matter to them. Ego gets in the way like this, and the Brahmans didn't realize the injustice they were doing. Hindus who converted later on believed the stories to be true. They don't even have any teachings, they are just stories. This is how people came to know Gommatesha as Ganesha, and Adinath as Shiva.

"Gommat" means "the bull," and "esha" is the "leader." It means that after Adinath left his body, Gommatesha became the leader of the bulls. All of the monks were in his hands. It means, after Shiva, Ganesha was the leader. "Gan" means "the group." Gommatesha and Ganesha are the same person. Hindus distorted the truth to hide their names and their teachings. Adinath became Shiva, and Gommatesha became Ganesha. Hindus were only trying to re-establish themselves, but in that, they didn't do justice to the real history and that is wrong. They could have kept the purity of Adinath but they didn't do it. Before the 8th century Hinduism had more truth. They were following Adinath's teachings then, along with all the other Tirthankaras.

When the Hindus became powerful they didn't care about the truth

44

anymore. Why would they want to know? Do Catholics want to know that karmic theory and incarnation theory used to be in their teachings? No one wants to know that any other faith exists. Everyone is in their own box and they will never get out unless they begin to see the truth. Catholics say they are the truth, and that's what Hindus think about themselves, too. They don't want to know the real truth. Buddhism was kicked out of India and Jains had a stronghold already, so the Hindus started to think they wanted to be the only ones.

Hindu is a very new word. Their idea is that it comes from the Sindhu civilization; after a long period of time it became Hindu. S in Sindhu, became an H. Sindhu became Hindu. I don't say Hindu culture, I say Indian culture instead. There are many religions in the Indian culture: Jainism, Buddhism, Sanaatan Dharma, Vaishnavism, and many more. But they began to call everyone Hindu. Hindu is not a religion, but a combination of many religions. Now people think Jains and Buddhists come from Hinduism. No one wants to know the history. Whoever gets stronger, that's who writes the history. It's always distorted.

Ganesha as we know him today is an example of this. His statues are all over the world, but he was not born with an elephant head, the way that Hindus depict him. Ganesha was the first son of Shiva, who lived on Mt. Kailash, and was born as a normal boy. There are many popular stories about him in Hindu and Indian mythology but they are full of contradictions. Indian mythology says that he was never even born. The popular story is that his mother Parvathi created him.

One day, Parvathi wanted to take a bath, but there were no bathrooms like we have these days with doors and privacy. You would take baths in an open area. So she was thinking, "No one is here. What if a stranger comes while I'm bathing?"

She rubbed her hands and there was a little dirt that came off her

45

hands. That dirt became Ganesha after it fell to the ground and she put her power into it. He was a very handsome man. So, according to Hindu mythology Ganesha was never born. He asked his mother, "What should I do for you?"

Parvathi told him to watch out for strangers and not let anyone come near because she was taking a bath. Ganesha was busy looking out around the area and protecting his mother when suddenly Shiva appeared. He saw someone standing near his home on Kailash.

"Who are you?"

And Ganesha asked, "Who are you?"

He said, "I am Shiva."

"I am Ganesha, Parvathi's son."

"I don't have any sons."

Ganesha told Shiva that he couldn't go any further because his mother was taking a bath. Shiva became angry with Ganesha and when he was stopped again, he cut Ganesha's head off. He went further and Parvathi was shocked, asking what happened to Ganesha. Shiva told that he had killed him and Parvathi said that she wanted him to be alive again. This is the way the story goes. Parvathi said she wanted him alive right now, no matter what. Shiva wanted to try and put his head back on but he couldn't find it anywhere. He went and ordered his army, called *gana*, to bring any head that fits on the boy's body. Nothing was fitting right. Finally in the forest they found a baby elephant and they brought its head and it fit perfectly. In the story it's said that Shiva put pranic-force in his body and he became Ganesha again. That is the story and now people are believing this is the real thing, the truth. This story is not the truth.

If Parvathi has so much power to make a boy from dirt, how could she not bring him back to life after his head was cut off? Shiva is known as a god in Hindu mythology, but he doesn't know who Ganesha is, that he's his own son, or that Parvathi made the boy. The story has many contradictions. If this Shiva was even real, he would know these things. He seems to be very angry in the story; would a god act this way, cutting off their own son's head?

The secret is that Ganesha – Gommatesha – was born spiritual. His body was very strong, and since the day he was born he was a very spiritual person. In order to be a parent or family member of a Tirthankara, that soul has to have a lot of qualities and be along their path already because the moment of enlightenment is not far for them – maybe the same life, or just several more. Gommatesha was always in his spiritual practices, always into his sadhana. He had two main teachings that he shared. They became so popular, and it's the reason why he is widely worshipped, even if the people worshipping him don't know the reasons. Whoever will teach about these things will be very popular, anyway, but he was the first intelligent young boy. Adinath even said that Gommatesha would be remembered more than him. And it's true, all of the Indian culture worships Ganesha before Shiva.

In those days there was no writing system. Everything had to be remembered and passed on to other people, and what he was teaching was very beautiful. He was teaching that you had to keep harmony between humans and animals. Sometimes animals are even more important than humans. On this planet there is a balance, and if the animals disappear the planet will be out of balance and the people will no longer be able to survive here. Gommatesha's devotees were thinking how they could keep his teachings alive, so they made a statue that was half-human and half-elephant. This way, if there was some kind of natural disaster, and since statues can survive a long time, whoever finds it in the future might understand the message of his teachings if they think deeply about it. We need his teachings very much today. We are killing animals. Killing animals means we are inviting many troubles on this planet. We should be filling ourselves with love and creating balance on this planet, but instead we are stuck in suffering because of this killing.

Ganesha's second teaching is very important. If we follow it this planet will be incredibly peaceful. Once a year, there is a big celebration in India – it's a tradition. They worship all the statues and the householders sing *bhajans*, or devotional songs, about Ganesha. In the evening before sunset, they do *visergen*; they throw all the statues in the ocean or river. All day they worship him as a god and then throw him in the water. Mostly the statues are clay so they don't create any pollution or trouble in the water. In India they don't know why they are even following this tradition. They are so blind I cannot believe it. They lost the real teachings from him: forget the attachment. This is what Gommatesha was teaching. Forget your attachment to people, to animals, or any things. Even if you have attachment to God, then you will never realize God. So throw it out after worshipping. That is an important teaching from Gommatesha. You have to go beyond this attachment. It's the biggest blockage in human life. If we cannot detach ourselves we will be deep in this world, wandering here and there and never thinking about spiritual growth.

First, create and keep harmony between humans, animals and all of nature. Second, don't even have attachment to God; otherwise you will not reach to God. This is why Ganesha is worshipped all over the world.

TIRTHANKARA SHRI PARSHVANATH

You know that the chakra system is a system of ancient teachings, but do you know where it came from? Most people think it came from Hinduism, or yogis or Chinese medicine. Yes, they were yogis, but not the kind that are known today. Yoga has become very polluted, and if you go to India looking for the true yogi, you might not find one. The truth has been forgotten, but I am revealing here the real chakra system, which is coming from the Samanic system of the Tirthankaras' teachings. The first kundalini master was *Parshvanath*, and he happened to be in the Jain system approximately 2,900 years ago. Notice I said Jain system and not Jain religion; they are two different things. The Jain system consists of practical techniques, like the chakra system, which help you grow spiritually, while the Jain religion is focused more on beliefs and rituals that are divided among multiple sects. Parshvanath is how we remember him today, but in his time he was called *Paasnaha*, because the language was different. He was the 23rd Tirthankara, born in Varanasi, India, and a historical figure whose palace ruins from before he renounced still remain today.

You cannot find his teachings today because they were lost. How did they become lost? What happened was there was no writing system in those days, and on top of that, Parshvanath didn't speak in a poetic language. It means that when something is spoken poetically it's easier to memorize and can be understood well. It's important because people were slower in that time and had a less-developed mind than we have today. They couldn't learn things as quickly, or grasp the deep meaning right away. They had to think about it again and again. Without poetic words it was difficult to remember his teachings and conserve them. There are just a few in the Jain sutra, the *Isibhasiyam Sutra*, but they are not his full system.

In the Isibhasiyam Sutra, he was called *Arhat Paasnaha*. "Arhat" means "enlightened one." He was teaching *chaturyam* – the four vows. After Parshvanath there were always five vows, but you will see why. The first vow of the chaturyam is *ahimsa* – nonviolence. Second is *satya* – truthfulness. Third is *asteya* – non-stealing. And the fourth is *aparigraha*; – non-possession. These vows are important to understand, but you have to go very deep into them. Since Mahavira's time, about 300 years after Parshvanath, there has been *mahavrata*, the five great vows. It seems like one vow is missing from Parshvanath's chaturyam. In those days women were considered a possession, so there was no need of the fifth vow, *brahmacharya*, which loosely translates to celibacy. It was included in aparigraha, non-possession, which would create some confusion later on between Parshvanath's last remaining devotees and Mahavira's monks. Brahmacharya is considered to be celibacy now, but it is not the right word. The real meaning of brahmacharya is that the one who takes this vow when they become a monk never takes their focus away from God, or from awakening their soul. They don't let anything distract them, take them astray from their path or waste their energy. So it doesn't just apply to abstaining from sex, it includes anything that doesn't help the person go deep into their consciousness and realize enlightenment. That is the real meaning of brahmacharya, but like most of the Tirthankaras' teachings, it has been forgotten or distorted.

Mahavira spoke mostly in a beautiful and poetic way. That's why many of his teachings are still known today, because they were memorized easily and recorded by the people. Also, he lived a little closer to our time and they had some writing then; Parshvanath's time didn't have that. All the Tirthankaras teachings are mostly lost because of their time period not having the system of writing and recording history, and many things were happening on the planet. A master can access the teachings because they know them already. Their knowing is the same, but someone has to ask, or maybe they won't say anything about it at all. Chakras are just how the energy works in the body. If someone becomes enlightened, they will understand that energy, but nobody asked any of the other Tirthankaras about it, only Parshvanath. Mahavira's teachings were a totally different system, and it attracted many people. He had different karmas to burn, so he had to go about it in a different way than Parshvanath. He was teaching renunciation more, to leave everything and be on the spiritual path. Even your own clothes. If you can do that, sitting naked in winter and summer, then you can tolerate anything in the world. People try to do it now, but today we cannot survive it because our bodies are weaker than that period of time. People were more attracted to the difficult way of sadhana. They lived in big open areas and there are huge mosquitoes there. They would sit in meditation and not worry about the bugs biting them. It can be very painful. There were five other teachers in Mahavira's time and they tried to show that they were better than him. It was like a competition, but Mahavira didn't get involved in it because he was the Tirthankara; he didn't care to show off anything. There was a monk who was not on the right path, his name was *Goshalak,* and his hair was full of lice. When the lice left his hair he would pick them up and put them all back onto his head. He said it was their home there. People were so mesmerized because they thought he didn't even have attachment to his own body. These kind of people were alive, like in our time now there are people like this, too, trying to show off. Maybe they don't live the same way, but they try to show they are popular. All these five people competing had robust personalities and tried to show off that they were good monks. Nobody was interested in learning about the chakras and the way their bodies worked. They wanted more visible things like renunciation and austerities, and many tried to show it off. *Gautama Siddhartha*, popularly known today as Buddha, was one of these five, and he couldn't understand how Mahavira had so many people going to him for initiation or just to be in his presence, so he sent his own disciples to listen to his lectures. Afterward, he would use Mahavira's words in his own lectures to try and attract more people to him. He is not like how Buddhists today think he was; he wanted to get a lot of respect.

Common people who remembered the teachings would eventually die off, and the Shramanas, the monks and nuns, lived away from central areas and went through a lot of harsh things during their practices. They would die in droughts, because times happened when there was no food available.

More or less, all poetic things are remembered, but I still consider that in Jain sutras, which mostly consist of Mahavira's teachings, there is no 100% guarantee in it that it's the truth. A lot of things are true in them, but if you take any kind of scripture or book that's considered holy, and say from A to Z that everything is right, then you are in a dilemma. Many things are lost. Writing started on a larger scale about 150 years after Mahavira was gone. Even though a lot of his teachings are available, more were still lost. The *Digambara* sect of Jains believes that all of Mahavira's teachings were lost, so they consider the sutras of the *Shvetambara* sect all false. Everything false. They don't look at themselves first. Their idea is that in the 8th century, *Kundakundacharya* had the ability to go to Tirthankaras, such as *Simandhar Swami*, on other planets and afterwards wrote the Digambara books from their teachings. They consider they have the only right teachings because of that Acharya. If he had that kind of power why didn't he just sit in meditation and go deep into his consciousness? Digambara sutras are all similar to Shvetambara sutras, and they are newer, too. Historically, Shvetambara books are the oldest. Poetic language was important in these periods of time. Maybe just the chakra activation sounds remained because they're small sounds and people remembered them more easily.

It happened occasionally that a monk was highly intelligent, a scholar kind of, and knew a lot of the teachings by memory. Sometimes they would share them with many other monks if they happened to visit them, but sometimes they would not even have contact with anyone, so when they eventually died the knowledge went with them. A lot of monks who knew Mahavira's teachings died like this. Droughts happened in 12-year cycles. Maybe there is now 10% of truth in the Jain sutras, but even that is a very big part of truth. You can learn many things from that 10% which can take you onto the path. Students of the Tirthankaras were carrying on the teachings and the system of society was changing, language was changing and the planet was changing. Somehow the sects continued but maybe the new monks didn't have the same experience or knowledge.

After Parshvanath became Siddha and merged with all the other liberated souls, there was one group of monks left who were following his chakra system and spiritual teachings. It happened 250 years after he was gone, and Mahavira was now alive. *Keshishramana* was the main monk of Parshvanath's sect of several hundred monks. They never met

Parshvanath, but they were following his teachings. They were staying in the city of Shraavasti and went out to collect alms one day, and on the way came across another group of monks. Keshishramana and his monks wore colorful clothes made of whatever patches they were given, and the other monks were all naked; no clothes at all. Gautam, also known as *Indrabhuti*, was the leader of these naked monks and the chief disciple of the 24th Tirthankara, Mahavira. Both groups exchanged their views of what they were doing and they suddenly were confused. Parshvanath was a Tirthankara, and those monks had taken four vows and wore clothing, and Mahavira is a Tirthankara now, and his monks took five vows and didn't wear any clothing. All the monks had a lot of doubts and decided to have a meeting to discuss the differences. Gautam was talking for Mahavira's monks, and Keshishramana was talking for Parshvanath's monks.

They discussed many things, including whether or not to wear clothing. Gautam was saying that Tirthankaras renounce everything, so why don't you be naked? In the end they compromised to wear white clothing as an option. Some of Mahavira's monks remained naked, but most of them dressed in white, including Gautam. In that time it was just a small piece of cloth they wrapped around, not a full covering. They compromised because then they will all look alike, and nobody wore white in that time, not even any Hindus. This way they would be recognized that they are following the Samanic system and people can find them to ask questions. Many monks disagreed and remained naked. It didn't matter to them; they were all equal still. If they wore white or went naked it didn't matter; neither was better than another. This was long before the Digambara sect started in Jainism. Digambara means "sky-clad," and they go completely naked, still today. There was not even the word "Digambara" when this meeting between the monks took place. They didn't have ego about it like the monks do today. After they decided to wear the white, you still had to bow to your senior monks even if you had decided to stay naked, or vice versa. They felt they were all equal; they were all on the same path. Wearing clothes or not wearing clothes makes no difference to your soul. Today, Digambara monks are going the wrong way. They think if you're not naked then you are not the real monk. They are fully ignorant. But Gautam was very wise and had a lot of vision for the future. He was a naked monk when the meeting took place, but realized it would be more difficult for monks to go into cities in the future if they were not clothed, among other troubles. Right away he began wearing white. Mahavira, being very democratic, didn't have a problem with it. He said if you want to wear white then wear white, but it didn't matter to him; he would remain as he had been without clothes. Digambara monks today have the idea that you have to be naked to reach to enlightenment. It means a tiny piece of thread is stronger than their own soul if it will really block their liberation. Monks used to live in forests and were starting to come into the cities. How many people would go into the forest when times changed and society became busier? Maybe one or two students. If you're wearing clothing you can go to the city. Jain teachings spread all over India because of Gautam.

No Digambara and no Shvetambara sects existed then, not even the words. They were all disciples of Mahavira. They ate the same, once a day, went around together, and sat together. If any of the monks were staying far away from a town or city, they would have to leave early in the morning, because it took time to walk. By the time they got there people were eating lunch, and families in those days lived all together. Sometimes it was 20 or 30 people in one house. They all cooked and ate together. When they finished eating lunch, the monks would arrive and families would give them the food they had cooked for their families. At night it was too dark to go out anyway, and on the way there was the possibility you might hurt yourself or harm insects and other things if you didn't see them, so monks didn't eat after dark. They didn't use fire in those days, and there was no system of electricity like we have today. No matter if they were clothed or naked they all went together. Over a long period of time they separated into two traditions: Shvetambara (clothed) and Digambara (naked) traditions.

All the monks merged together and became disciples of Mahavira as a result of the meeting. They were asking a lot of questions and it seems like they knew some of the chakra system. Even though it was 250 years since Parshvanath, Keshishramana was asking to Gautam how to get the mind to stop resisting all the time. Maybe they had forgotten most of the actual system of chakras, but the mind will bother you a lot if your sixth and seventh chakras are not balanced, so it seems like they had some experience. The way Gautam answered was beautiful. He told Keshishramana that if you have a reign in your hand, no matter how wild the horse is, then you can discipline the mind to take you where you want to go. He used the reign as a metaphor to describe discipline such as, tapas (fasting), meditation, and *japa* (repeating mantras). They were still carrying the ideas of the chakra system but not clearly. I am reviving it today, because I remember in my past life I was with Parshvanath, so the system is not completely lost. He was teaching about kundalini, and making your body healthy, otherwise you cannot awaken your soul. Jains are so ignorant still – Digambara and Shvetambara both. They keep his statue in the same way since his time but they don't think about his teachings at all. They worship him without knowing. Many Jains make his statue with a hood of a thousand snakes around his head. There are not a thousand chakras in the body, but they keep adding and adding snakes on his statue because they don't know what it represents.

These are some of the ways that Parshvanath's teachings were lost, and the same thing happens with the other Tirthankaras. He is even the most popular Tirthankara still today, but no one has his teachings. The monks initiated by him were the last of the Nath sect. It was just part of his name, so his monks were known by that. They were also called *Parshvaapatyaka* – the children of Parshvanath.

Parsh means, "side." Jains believe that when his mother was pregnant, she noticed snakes passing by her side one day, so they called him Parsh. It can be *Paras*, too, or *Paas*. In Prakrit there is no word Parsh. A paras is a stone that is not found anymore, but if you have it you can touch iron to the stone and it will turn to gold. It used to be common to find them. It's more likely that this was the meaning, because in his time the sounds in Prakrit were different and Parsh didn't exist. Parsh is from the Sanskrit language and became a popular name for him later. He was actually called Paasnaha when he was living.

If you go to India and ask a Jain why he has the seven-hooded snake over his head they will tell you that it's his symbol, but they don't really know why. Do Jains even wonder where it came from? They think it's just a symbol. They think that all the Tirthankaras are born with the symbol. Adinath's society was very innocent and loyal and the bull represents that. It's why Jains call him Rishabhdeva, the bull. There is one story about Parshvanath that is known by all the Jains. There was a monk named *Kamatha*, and he was known for doing austerities. Long before Parshvanath renounced the world, when he was a young boy, his mother wanted to go and see Kamatha because word spread that he was doing some kind of ritual and sitting with big fires all around him. Kamatha was a monk but he had a lot of ego; he wanted to show how much he could tolerate by sitting so close to the fires. People could not believe how amazing it was and they came to pay respect from all over. Parshvanath went with his mother and saw that all the people were mesmerized. Because Parshvanath had avadhi jnana, he could see there were two snakes trapped inside one of the logs that Kamatha had placed in the fire. He went in front of Kamatha and it made him so angry. Kamatha was thinking that this boy in front of him was jealous of his popularity and wanted to ruin his show. Parshvanath told him why not cut open the log and see for yourself the snakes that are burning to death in your fire. They were burned so badly that they were about to die, so Parshvanath recited the Namokar mantra for them and they passed away peacefully. When the snakes died they were born on an angel planet because they were in such positive thoughts from hearing the mantra. They became the angels *Dharnendra* and *Padmavati*. Angels are not what people think, flying around with wings. They rarely leave their own planets and they have a limited life. Even though it can be a very long life, it is still limited. Later when Kamatha died he was born on one of the lowest angel planets. He saw Parshvanath, as an adult, meditating in the standing position one day, because all angels have avadhi jnana and can see things certain distances away from their planet. Remembering what had happened in his last life, he still held anger against Parshvanath and wanted to kill him. While Parshvanath was standing, Kamatha brought many bad things to him, but he remained unaffected in meditation. Finally Kamatha decided he would make a flood and drown him. The rain was so much that the water was building and slowly reached Parshvanath's knees, then higher and higher until it was up to his mouth. Dharnendra and Padmavati saw it happening and remembered that Parshvanath had recited the Namokar mantra for them when they were in the fire. They came to his aid and lifted him from the water so he didn't drown. This is the belief of Jains; it's a popular story. If you see a statue of Parshvanath you will see that Padmavati is with him, too. But it still doesn't answer the question about the seven snakes over his head. Even though the story has the snakes, there are only two; why would his statue have seven?

I consider Parshvanath the first kundalini master, because he was the first Tirthankara who talked about chakras and how the body works in this way. All Tirthankaras have the same knowing, but they will only talk about something if they are asked. None of the other Tirthankaras were asked about chakras until Parshvanath. The chakra system started with him, 2,900 years ago. Many things affect our chakras because they are in our body; if our organs are working improperly, or we have headaches, it's all related to chakras. In his time, the people were very curious about their bodies. They wanted to know how their systems worked and how they could make their bodies healthy and go into deep meditation. They were curious like snakes are. Parshvanath's symbol has two meanings. The seven-hooded snake represents his main teachings: the chakra system and how to wake up your kundalini, and it also represents the curiosity of the people who lived in the society. Why are there seven snakes? Because in the human body there are seven main chakras. This is the truth behind his symbol. His students were wise and knew that one day, things would be forgotten, so they thought if they created this symbol on his statue that people would understand it was representing the seven chakras and giving the message to make your body pure and full of energy for the spiritual path. It's a beautiful teaching, but completely forgotten even by the Jains who worship him so much.

Our history is not accurate because it doesn't mention the first kundalini master anywhere. Even though all over India, and even outside of India, his statues are in many places, nobody knows his teachings. Parshvanath's teachings were very practical. I liked him a lot. They were not like Mahavira's teachings that you had to think about and try to understand. Anything practical is good because if you do it, then you will get the result. Spirituality is practicality. If you do your sadhana and put all your effort into it, then you will start to unfold all of the layers inside you and understand the deeper things. You don't have to think about it, just do the practical things. Soul is beyond the mind, so thinking too much about it won't take you there anyway. Even the word "spirituality" cannot contain spirituality; you must experience it to know its vastness.

The kundalini awakening is important for the human body, because you will feel heavy and dark otherwise. Depression will come and keep you down, and you'll be restless or sad, living with a foggy cloud around your mind and unable to see things clearly or be passionate for your life. Kundalini is the energy in your body that makes you healthy and you'll be able to go on the spiritual path. Parshvanath was talking about these things, how the body is affected and what you can do to balance your energy centers.

It is really something special to be with a Tirthankara. They won't speak unless you ask; otherwise people just come and sit silently around him. Peace is felt so strongly, and your body feels so light that you will even forget your questions sometimes. You just want to sit there for a while and feel peace. Once in a while someone will ask something, and whoever is sitting near can hear the response from the Tirthankara. I remember people were coming to Parshvanath and asking, "Through this body, how can we be awakened?"

Parshvanath would answer briefly. He said that if you change the oil in the body, you clear the toxins out and get stronger to do sadhana and burn your karma. These days it's understood what changing the oil means; we know about cars and machines so we understand the meaning. There was a difficulty in understanding Parshvanath's teachings because of the way he spoke. I mentioned he didn't use poetic language, but he sometimes would say things that were not known. An enlightened person can see a lot of things, so he mentioned oil sometimes but no one knew about changing the oil, they didn't get the meaning. When he answered about the energy in our bodies he started saying, "chakra;" wheel.

When you're in the presence of the Tirthankara you don't want to talk. In their presence all of your questions are lost, they're dissolved. They don't usually demonstrate techniques but they will explain it so people can get it. Parshvanath would recite the sounds of the chakras just one time if someone asked, and they would practice it. Or, he would describe a posture to put their body into, a yoga posture. He might sit a certain way and people understood they had to do the same thing. There are many postures not known in Hatha yoga. Someone would ask him how to open the first chakra and Parshvanath would sit a certain way. He might show someone else a different technique if that's what they needed. He never spoke in detail, only briefly. But when an enlightened person speaks one sentence and whoever is listening remains quiet, it means they have to say it again to help the person understand.

Historically, all of these things have been lost, but a master can connect with them through meditation and share them, even if they're wiped off the Earth and all of the books are lost. In India they don't think, "Why is Parshvanath's statue different from all the others?" If the snakes are just a symbol, why put it over his head? All the other Tirthankaras' statues have just a little symbol below where they sit, so why put his on his head? Parshvanath was the only one teaching the kundalini system in detail: what sounds affect different chakras and heal the body, how colors work in the body and raising your intention to elevate your energy. All of these things he was teaching to people, and they were very practical things.

The *Nath Sampradai*, the nath sect, was created after his name later on by the monks and nuns following his system, but even before that, the nath originally came from Adinath. There were other Tirthankaras with "nath" in their names; Mallinath and Ajitanath are two examples. I can tell you that in the remains of the Sindhu civilization they found a statue of a monk sitting in a meditative state. It's believed that the statue is of Adinath. The Samanic system, the universal spiritual teachings, was flourishing in the Sindhu area. Tirthankaras didn't go to that place, they stayed mostly in west, central and north India towards Nepal, Tibet, and up to Delhi, but many monks travelled to share their teachings. Sindhu is now located in Pakistan. Hindus believe the statue to be of Shiva, but the real Shiva is Adinath. In the Hindu's mind, Shiva has a snake around his neck and he dances. They call it *Nataraja*, the king of dance, but the real thing was the dancing posture from the Samanic system. If you stay in that yoga posture it creates so much energy in you.

A Tirthankara never creates a sect or even the Tirtha. Jains are completely in the dark in this aspect. The Tirtha happens because of all of the monks and nuns, but the Tirthankara doesn't set it up. It just happens. All the monks follow what the Tirthankara does; they try to imitate them. Even though the Tirthankara always says not to imitate, but to be natural, to be yourself, they still tried to. That becomes their system. If the Tirthankara meditates, the monks begin to meditate. If they're sitting peacefully, not eating, then the monks do the same. That's how fasting started. They understood to do the same, and after some time they had experience in going without food, and sometimes without both food and water. If a bug sits on their body and they leave it alone, then the monks would do the same thing.

The term "Tirthankara" always existed since Adinath. We always called them that. Tirthankara Shri Adinath, or Tirthankara Shri Parshvanath that's how you would call them. Around them the Tirtha forms. The four Tirthas are the Shramanas (monks), Sadhvis (female

monks), *shravakas* and *shravikas* (male and female householders). The householders are still living in the societal life, but they dedicate their life to the spiritual teachings of the enlightened ones. The Tirtha means that wherever they go to, all of the people's hearts change. This is the *Jangam Tirtha*, the moveable Tirtha. The Jangam Tirtha is wherever the Shramanas and Sadhvis are meditating, traveling, or teaching. The other Tirtha is the *Sthavar Tirtha* – a place where a Tirthankara spends time, or the place where they achieved enlightenment, or where they leave their body later on and become liberated. You can bring that energized soil and water and establish a miniature Tirtha, like at Siddhayatan. Wherever Parshvanath left his body is considered a Tirtha. Wherever Mahavira or Mallibai achieved enlightenment is a Tirtha. Mallibai was the 19th Tirthankara and the only Tirthankara to have a female body in this time period. The Digambara Jain sect considers it was actually a male named Mallinath, but they reject the truth. Someone even asked Mahavira once if it was a male or a female and he replied that Mallibai was female. To have a female or male body as a Tirthankara doesn't make a difference. When you are in that state of knowing you are beyond your body, just living inside of it. Anyone can reach enlightenment, there's no restriction to a female or male body, and anyone who is teaching this is in illusion.

Parshvanath's monks were mostly based in west India, south India and Gujarat – northwest India. That was their stronghold, and still today. In south India there is almost nothing now, except Digambaras because of the Bahubali statue. It's the only statue like that in the entire world – a 57 foot tall monolithic statue. Parshvanath's teachings are popular in those areas now because he was roaming around there with his monks. They had a lot of impact in the society; all the kings were following him. He was teaching to make the body divine, a temple. Temples in those days were different but had a similar idea. You don't take dirt into the temple, so why would you put dirt in your body? Make it clean and pure so divinity can enter in you. It is all around you, waiting for that moment, but you miss the opportunities. All of his teachings were practical things. Mahavira doesn't seem to be a practical teacher at all, but his understanding is marvelous, incomparable. I prefer practical. Theory has its own value, too, if you understand on the deepest level, but there wasn't anyone like that in Parshvanath's time. If somebody could speak a language, even unclearly, they were considered the highest. Education didn't exist, there was no system to learn like how we have today.

Tirthankaras will teach whatever the people need at the time, because that's what the people will ask about. Their questions were more practical. If you find his statues anywhere, they show him in kayotsarga, a unique standing position for meditation, more than Mahavira's statues. It was more popular in Parshvanath's time, and he taught many secrets about it. It's not that you just stand there. No, you have to do it in a certain way to create the energy. Most of the time Parshvanath stood in kayotsarga position.

Nearby the Muslim pilgrimage place, Mecca, there used to be a statue of Parshvanath standing in kayotsarga. In that area people were following the Samanic teachings and yogic system, and there were big statues to remember him. This was before the Islam religion started. When Islam became popular there, they began destroying the statues by first cutting all of the heads from them. People still came to see them and when power came into the hands of a new group, they thought the statues looked bad without their heads and decided to smooth them completely. They sanded the Parshvanath statue so the arms weren't visible next to the body, because in kayotsarga you stand with your arms right alongside your body touching your hands against your thighs. It was entirely smoothed out into a big stone with no features remaining. Later they regretted destroying them, but today when you go to Mecca they still carry the same tradition. Some of it was added later on, but the original still remains. Keshishramana and Gautam merged their *sanghas*, their orders, and began wearing white, and even today the Muslims still wear white when they go to the Ka'aba where they keep the Black Stone. You have to take a vow to not kill anything and have pure thoughts when you're there; Islam doesn't have any of this in their teachings. When you leave the site you can later go and sacrifice an animal, but not while you're there. You go around the stone three times minimum. The tradition never changed. Hindus believe it is Shiva, because he had a dark skin tone and his statues are mostly like that, but he wasn't known to practice the standing position so it doesn't make sense. It seems like it was Parshvanath because he had a similar color skin and was always in kayotsarga. By the time the stone was smoothed out, it was so popular that all the Jain business people were giving money there before Islam took over. Many Jain pilgrimages were run by Muslims, even within India. There was a period when Muslim kings were ruling over India. There is history like that. After the campus in Mecca, some leave to go and sacrifice animals. They can't do it when they're inside, but afterwards they forget about the vow of nonviolence and having pure thoughts. Pilgrims go to throw stones at the wall, what they call, "Stoning the Devil." That devil is nothing. When people would visit the Parshvanath statue they would throw stones; it was symbolic. The devil is a bad guy, right? It represents Kamatha. Jains started that, though in those days they weren't known as Jains. They threw the stones at Kamatha because he tried to drown Parshvanath while he was in meditation. The tradition has not changed since the very beginning. It is just a matter of research. Muslims need to learn how the stone came to be there, but they don't want to hear anything. When something is popular no one wants to hear the truth anymore. The truth is that it was a statue of

Parshvanath many years ago.

Parshvanath was widely known in his time and is widely known now. More than any other Tirthankara, among the Jains even. He used to say that if you can make your body pure and divine like a temple, it's the best thing you can do. God comes only into the pure. Nowadays it seems like temples and churches are not pure, but in those days temples were a little different. There is a system to make your body pure, and you have to follow through all the steps. Parshvanath was familiar with many yogic techniques. He went through the system. It is very difficult to do this; you can never put anything impure into this body, such as alcohol, fish, meat and eggs, all of which deteriorate your body and invite toxins. With a lot of practice your body becomes pure in such a way that it cannot even tolerate these toxic things in its system. They will make you very sick, because your body is light and pure, very healthy, and it will shock your body too much. Parshvanath's chakra system is full of beautiful teachings that people need to know about. For thousands of years this system was taught, and it's very easy to follow. If your chakras are very balanced, your life will transform. Your life will be very joyful. If you have these things, maybe one day when a monk, saint or a spiritual teacher tells you just one little thing, you might begin to think about how you can improve yourself and raise your energy up. You will feel your body is becoming lightened. In India, the people who follow Jain teachings have forgotten the true system behind the teachings.

What Parshvanath was teaching was extraordinary. He was the first kundalini master, because he was the only Tirthankara to share the practical system of taking toxins out of your body and raising your energy, your kundalini. This is what the people in his time were curious about. When your body becomes pure and your seven chakras are balanced, you're almost in bliss.

"Parshvanath's leshya system is actually the chakra system."

Parshvanath was teaching what was known as *leshyas.* Jains today know of leshyas, but the original meaning is lost. When Gautam brought Keshishramana and his monks to be initiated under Mahavira, all of the teachings they remembered were merged and they changed because they mixed with Mahavira's. Because Mahavira was living a totally different system and people were different, they were not as interested in practical things. Instead they became more theoretical and tried to deepen their understanding and go deep into their souls. As far as the chakra system goes, Jains don't know it started with Parshvanath because they were known more as leshyas in those days, not chakras.

Leshya is very important to understand. The meaning of leshya is, "*Kashaaya yoga ranjita leshya.*" *Kashaaya yoga* means when your body, mind and speech are mixed with your intentions. The four kashaayas are: anger, ego (pride), deceit and greed. *Ranjita* means it is colored by those things; it's not pure. That is called *leshya.* If you go to the higher leshya, the color is taken out; it means the intention is more pure and the kashaayas are less. The higher your intention, the less color, like removing dirt from water.

What intention do you have? Intention is important, because whatever intention you have, combined with the actions by your body and activities in your mind disrupt the flow of your energy and collect karma. This energy creates all the colors in your body that belong to the different chakras.

You can transform your leshya, your intention, from low to high. It is up to you. When there is no intention anymore, you can't collect karma. Even though your body and thoughts are involved in doing different actions, there is no longer any leshya, no intention, so you can't collect karma, you just go through the remaining karma until nothing is left and you are liberated. Let me give you an example. Suppose you're walking and you don't have an intention to harm any living being, like stepping on a worm or insect, and suddenly it comes under your foot; you feel bad because you were paying attention to not harm them, but it happened anyway. Or, you're driving and an animal jumps out in the road. You swerve to try and save it, but the animal moves at the same time out of fear and you end up hitting them anyway. You tried to protect the animal from dying, but in doing so it was killed anyway. That is a pure intention. Always having a pure intention will burn your karmas. If your intention is, "I am going to try and save this animal, so I will get good karma," then you will get good karma instead of burning karma. This is known as *punya*: doing actions in order to collect good karma for your future. It means you want the good result in your life. Many people practice this in India. The more karma you collect, either good or bad, it becomes dense like fog and covers your soul. The spiritual person wants to burn all of their karma to become free, not collect more. They learn spiritual practices and live in discipline in order to do so. When a person practices punya to get good results from their karma, it shows they're not balanced, because they don't want to go through difficult things. That is not a spiritual person. A spiritual person remains balanced during good and bad experiences.

There are some karmas that cannot be burned. These are called *Nikachita karma*. No matter how much effort is put, they will remain until the time comes for them to give you the result. If you put a lot of effort you can reduce the effect, but you can't burn them away completely like other karmas. Of course, if you don't put any effort at all then they will give you the worse result, according to the karma. Mahavira had to go through 12-and-a-half years of suffering because he had a lot of Nikachita karma. He wouldn't have gone through so much suffering if he didn't have those karmas.

Everyone has Nikachita karma. How can you collect it? Suppose somebody is a hunter. They already have the worst intention, and they're collecting a lot of karma for killing the animals. Deer, elephants, fish, birds, they are all living beings and experience fear and pain. The hunter shoots an animal, and right away they jump in the air and celebrate. So, the hunter did very badly and then they are proud of it. When you are so proud of yourself when doing bad things, you collect the Nikachita karma and have to go through the result one day.

It happens the opposite way, too. Suppose a high building is on fire. All the people are stuck on the 20th floor. I saw this in Delhi, India. No one could help because they were so high up. Police were there, but they were helpless. It was a bad situation and everyone was in a panic. No one could do anything. Thousands of people were there, but one guy didn't listen to anyone. He ignored the police and told people to do this and do that. They built a huge ladder on the roof of a lower building next to the high one. With the ladder they made a kind of bridge and it was wide enough for people to walk. He saved hundreds of people right in front of us. All of the people were busy talking about what to do and they didn't do it. This one guy got the idea and moved right away. He saved hundreds of people. By the time they put out the fire, only 2 or 3 stories burned. He did a very good thing and he wasn't even thinking about himself; he just saw the people and took action to help them. Until that point he was okay, but afterward, when everyone was safe on the ground, he jumped in the air and was smiling and celebrating how many people he saved. So, he will get the very good karma, but it is Nikachita karma because of his pride. He cannot burn it and will have to go through the result of it one day, even though it will be a very good result. This kind of karma keeps you trapped in the cycle of birth and death for a long time, because you have to wait for them to come on the surface; you can't do anything about it, only wait. You need five senses and a mind to collect these kind of heavy karmas. Because we have all the sensations of touch, sight, hearing, taste and smell available to us, we can experience things fully, all the pain and all the joy, too. Humans have the most developed mind. We're able to think, process, analyze, make decisions, be creative; it allows us to collect the heaviest karma, because we're supposed to know about what we're doing with all of these things available in our body. If we feel pain from something, we should know that maybe someone else might feel that pain also, or even a little bug. We can use our mind to decide not to make this pain for anything else, but we don't think this way.

But what about when our intention is always changing? One moment we might feel very good and help people all day without thinking about it, and then at night we become angry at something and our intention drops very low. Karma cannot touch the soul, because soul is shapeless, formless. The sun is always shining, right? Soul is the same way. Soul is surrounded by the clouds of karma. Karma is not touching the soul. The soul cannot see through the darkness because the karmas are so dark like thick clouds over many lifetimes of being collected. Sometimes the clouds are so thick in the sky that the sunlight can't pass through yet, but the sun is still millions of miles away from the clouds. In the same way, the soul is always shining like this, but it's weak and the karmas are too thick. The sun might die one day, maybe billions of years from now, but the soul never dies. So, if your intention is always changing, you will collect good karma in one moment and bad karma in the next moment. Soul is in the grip of karma when karmic particles are being attracted to you. It can't see through until the clouds can be removed. You burn them, or create wind, like a hurricane. That hurricane means going deep into your sadhana with your entire heart. You're completely present and aware in your spiritual practice with your whole being and nothing distracts you. It will create chaos inside you and the karmas will begin to move. To burn them you create fire by fasting with water, or fasting with nothing at all, sadhana, practicing austerities, and so on.

Karma is collected by our leshya, our intention. I will give a story to explain intention:

Six different people are out walking and come to a tree. It's a very hot day and this tree is creating a lot of shade. Suppose it's a mango tree, and they're very ripe. The first person to reach the tree has a very bad leshya – *Krishan* leshya. This is the lowest leshya. The first person says, "I want to collect all these fruits, but I want to collect them as soon as possible." So they cut the whole tree down. This is the lowest intention and collects a lot of karma; they want to get the fruit right away. Even though there are better ways, they still cut the whole tree down for the small fruits.

The second person comes and says, "I want to collect all these fruits and take them home. If I cut all the big branches of the tree, then I can pick up all the fruit when they land on the ground." Their intention is a little bit better, but still not very good. This is called *Neel* leshya.

The third person comes and also wants the mangoes. They think if they cut the medium branches and leave the bigger ones, they can pick the fruit when the branches come down and the tree is mostly okay. Still, they have a little better intention than the first and second person, but still the intention is low. This is called *Kapota* leshya.

Then the fourth person comes to the mango tree. They decide to just cut the smallest branches that are holding the mangoes. Their intention is higher. This called *Tejo* leshya.

The fifth one comes and thinks that it is better to climb the tree and shake the branches, because they don't want to harm the tree by cutting it down, or taking the branches off. This intention is called *Padma* leshya.

Then the last person comes and they lay out a huge blanket beneath the tree. They wait. The wind comes and all the ripe mangoes begin to fall down into the blanket. So this sixth person goes home with all the mangoes, like the others, but their intention is the purest, the *Shukal* leshya.

When you check how your intention is, you might find out which chakras are not active enough and why your kundalini is not rising. This is what Parshvanath was teaching 2,900 years ago. This is the message of his statue that his students created, but the Jains today are ignorant and don't want to see it. Statues are not meant to be worshipped, they are symbolic of spiritual teachings. They are going to stay in the dark in the Krishan leshya, but Parshvanath's teaching was to transform your leshya from Krishan up to Shukal. All the Jains need to be awakened. They worship his statues but refuse to hear the truth of his teachings. They have the treasure but they don't value it. If they begin to combine the leshyas with the chakras, all over the world the system will be spread. This system cannot be kept hidden in a little box. Even the scholars don't discover these things because they don't want to look in the right places.

PATAÑJALI AND YOGA

Most people consider the *Yoga Sutras* to be the first book on yoga, but this idea is wrong. I don't use the words written by Patañjali; I say they were compiled by Patañjali. Patañjali collected teachings and shared them in one book. This is the first book that became popular, and these days Patañjali is the most known, but he didn't write the sutras. Patañjali's time was a maximum of 2,850 years ago, so it shows he was after Parshvanath. The sutras are from around 800 B.C., and Parshvanath was living around 900 B.C. Some scholars think that the sutras were written in 850 B.C., but all of the scholars agree that they were between 800 and 850 B.C. – still fifty years after Parshvanath.

Patañjali was a marvelous person. What he did, he did a very good job. He had an idea that all of the teachings of the yogic system and from Parshvanath's system could be digested and made into one book. All the seeds were already there and he brought them together. Adinath was the first yogi, but has been forgotten, yet Patañjali is remembered and even called a master, or great sage. Westerners, Hindus and Jains, they need to understand this illusion, and see that Patañjali has nothing to do with yoga. Patañjali simply compiled a book to bring all the teachings in one place.

What he did was write them in short sentences, as sutras, so they were easy to remember. He was very intelligent, like a scholarly kind of person. He had a sharp mind and was good at dividing the steps of yoga separately. No one else would have thought to do it. There were a few other books like this, too. It was good to write beliefs like this so people could memorize them easily. They put a lot of things in one place, like trying to fill the whole ocean into one pot. At least he did a very good job, but they are not his teachings.

Patañjali was not a yogi or an ascetic, or even interested much in spirituality. He was just a simple, normal person who had a big desire to be famous. In the original sutras he even talked about himself, but they were lost after some time. He didn't practice the system. You can collect all the devotional songs or folk songs into one big book, but it doesn't mean you wrote them or know how to sing them. If Patañjali was a spiritual person he would be known as a yogi, but he's not. In India he is even known as a scholar. It seems like he didn't know what enlightenment meant, because otherwise he would have talked about it more in the sutras. Mostly he talked about *samadhi,* the last stage of yoga, but he didn't mention enlightenment. All of the discipline is good though. If it's practiced in society it will create good health and pure thoughts. Most of the sutras are about the disciplines, called *yama* and *niyama.* The dos and don'ts. They are coming from the Samanic system, which is why they're very similar to the vows that Jain monks take nowadays. He brought everything from the Samanic system. Instead of the four vows from Parshvanath's monks, he included five. He came after Parshvanath, so women were respected a little more, but still not as much as when the 24th Tirthankara Mahavira lifted women so high up in society.

It's unfortunate that the *Yoga Sutras* are a marvelous compilation, but people only practice yoga postures, *asanas*, more than anything.

Otherwise Patañjali's soul would be collecting a lot of good karma for inspiring the people in yoga today.

In those sutras, this is what he said about postures: "*Sthira sukham asanam.*" It means for your body to be in such a way that is steady and without tension. There are much better books about yoga postures, and they are in detail. Postures are just good for health. That's why they were created, so your body becomes healthy. Nobody follows yama and niyama, the first two steps that are the foundation of the spiritual path and are the most beneficial for you. You have to understand many teachings and be under great discipline, then come to yoga postures, then *pranayama* (breathing exercises), then *pratyahara* to look inside, then concentration and meditation, then you come to samadhi. These are the steps, but who follows them? Patañjali is praised by many people, yet according to him, yoga postures are not the whole of yoga, just one small part. Modern yoga teachers follow his book, yet they drink alcohol at the same time. They are eating meat and eggs, and many even use drugs. These people are considered yoga teachers? Are they really following the system that was compiled in the sutras, or are they just in illusion? Patañjali won't collect much good karma because yoga teachers are not straightened out; they're not teaching the right things, even if they claim to follow his book. His soul today, wherever it is, will still collect some good karma for inspiring people here and there, but if the majority straightened out and followed the discipline, which is mostly what the sutras are about, then he will get so much credit for it – so much good karma.

Even in India, a few famous yoga schools write that if you drink one or two cups of alcohol there's nothing wrong with that. These are not real yoga teachers. First, yoga teachers are supposed to be following the discipline and understanding; barely any teachers live this way and they claim to be yoga teachers or call themselves "yogis?" Shame on them. If you keep putting bad stuff in your body it doesn't matter how much practice you do. Yoga is becoming more of an exercise and that is wrong. It's not supposed to be exercise, it's supposed to be a mastery. You sit for a couple hours in one posture and gain mastery, not just one minute in lion posture. At least stay for 30 minutes in lion posture, then you will see how much energy it creates in your body.

If Westerners visit one time in India, and they see a sadhu, they are mesmerized and think, "Wow, they are in samadhi." They touch their feet and they come home and tell people they know what samadhi is. If those people can claim to know about it, what's wrong about Patañjali claiming to know samadhi? He could write, and a writer can share better than a yogi what the yogi experiences, because they can mesmerize people with their words. It doesn't necessarily mean they achieved that. Patañjali never even taught the sutras. He had no followers and no students, because he wasn't a teacher. He simply tried to use his writing ability to share the yoga teachings and get fame for himself.

It shows that he didn't achieve that state because he had many misunderstandings about yoga. He tried to interpret yoga into one line by writing, "*Yogaschchitta vriti nirodhah.*" *Chitta vriti* is all the constant changes going on in your mind. If you restrain them by controlling them that is called yoga; according to Patañjali, you have to control your mind. He is clear about it and that is totally wrong. Yoga is to understand the mind. If you understand the mind more, and don't try to control it at all, it will become your friend. The more you try to restrain it, the more it becomes your enemy. All these Hindu swamis following the *Yoga Sutra* are trying to control the mind, and they teach this to everyone. They see the mind as the main obstacle, so they try to control it. They make holes in their ears and put weights hanging from them, or stand on one leg all day or lie on thorns. They think these are austerities and will help them to overcome their minds. A lot of ignorant things like that are being done in India. They are torturing themselves and keeping themselves in more darkness. That is where his biggest statement went wrong. He could have said that yoga is when you are fully balanced. He got stuck interpreting the mind more. If you try to control the changes of the mind, they get even stronger, but if you try to understand them, they might dissolve one day. Dissolving the modifications of the mind is a better thing to describe yoga, but the way he wrote it is a wrong statement.

If you ask me the true definition of yoga, I will say, "*sahajyoga,*" just sit quietly. Let it happen, whatever happens. You just become a witness and watch what is happening. If you become that, the witness, you split in two ways. Your body and senses become separate. That is the only way to witness, otherwise you cannot do it. I can also call it "*layayoga,*" when you merge yourself the natural way. When you are into this state fully and sit quietly, you can go deeper and deeper. Some kind of rhythm picks up. "*Nadha;*" it means the sound. You begin to hear nadha. It's a beautiful sound, not like birds chirping. It's very beautiful. You have never heard that kind of sound in your whole life. That is supposed to be the definition of yoga.

In Jainism they define yoga totally different from Patañjali. They wrote in Jain texts that yoga is when the modifications of your mind, body and speech dissolve by understanding. At least they made a very good statement. In Patañjali's sutras he included a definition that is more controlling, and controlling doesn't make you liberated, or "*jivamukta,*" as Jains call it.

If people followed the first two steps of Patañjali's sutras, yama and niyama, they would have a better chance of being on the real path, but who wants to do it? Many people don't want to even do pranayama, so they jump to meditation and skip everything before it. You can't jump to meditation if you don't follow the system. You have to follow the discipline, clear the toxins out of your body; there are many things which keep a person from letting go of their mind and entering into the meditative state. It's not that you just decide to sit in a yoga posture and you are suddenly in meditation. No; you have to go through a lot of things. Most people do maybe one yama, practice postures and try to jump to meditation, and they don't understand why they're not getting anywhere. If you want to jump high, the chances are you will fall down. I know many yogis in India, and most of them are in jail. They tried to control their mind and it got so strong that they went crazy. Even though they might look like a yogi, they are not on the path at all. Yogis have a bad name these days. I was in Switzerland once when I met a temple priest. He's considered a yogi there among the people, but he told me that he is just a priest, that he has children and a family, but he wears those clothes and the people love it. He told me not to go to India with these white clothes on my body because the yogis in India are not taken seriously anymore. He said that when he goes to India, he changes his whole outfit and wears Western-style clothing. He doesn't want people to get an idea that he is a yogi. People are losing a lot of respect for yogis in India, because they're misdoing a lot of things; they have very bad behavior. But the monks and nuns are still respected highly.

Why do you think that everywhere today you can find yoga posture teachers who are not even spiritual? They are following teachings from ignorant yogis and misinterpreting books that they read. Nobody really wants to be truly spiritual these days. It is difficult to be on the spiritual path. People just want to pick and choose what fits their schedule and they think it will lead them somewhere? These posture teachers, which I call them, need to understand a lot of things before they can consider themselves a yoga teacher. First, they made teaching yoga postures into a profession; it's not supposed to be a profession. They rent the studios and try to make money and have a living by it. It's okay for those people who are just enjoying stretching their bodies and getting exercise, but it has polluted the real thing. Yoga was just a side-job. You have a main job and then a small thing on the side. Teaching others is a side-job. If it brings a little money that's fine, but don't depend on it. The Western students are doing something wrong, because they try to make it their main profession. When it became a main profession in the Western countries that's when it became polluted. Students are good, they want to learn about yoga and are attracted to the ideas, but if the teacher doesn't follow all the disciplines, how can they recommend other people to do it? The first step of yama is nonviolence. You have to be fully vegetarian. If you are not, how can you follow any of the steps past the first one? You cannot purify your body and mind by simply doing Hatha yoga postures. Of course, your body will be healthier than when you began, be less stiff, but even if you do postures every day, you will then go and put more pollution in your body with meat and alcohol, heavy foods and abusive substances. Some teachers in India are good, they try to follow the system, but yoga is not their main profession. They have other businesses and teach yoga in their free time. Bring yourself on the spiritual path and indulge your heart into sadhana before you think to teach other people about it.

These yogis are not really yogis in our time. They can give themselves their own name like *Gurunath, Yoginath, Yogiraj, Gururaj*; it shows that they don't want to be less than anybody else when they make a name like that. They're not following the real nath tradition. They're following the nath from the ninth-century Hatha yoga masters, *Matsyendranath* and *Gorakshanath*. Hatha yoga was already there since Adinath. Whatever Adinath started was simply repeated later on through the teachings. These "Yogirajs" and "Gururajs" belong to that kind of tradition. It's a branch of the original nath lineage, but it is a very distant branch. They became stuck into miracles and ego and forgot about awakening their soul to reach enlightenment. They try to change the shape of their body with *siddhis* (spiritual powers) and sit naked and harm their bodies. They're stuck and mesmerized by siddhis. They even say the same thing, but they don't know what it is. Parshvanath used to tell people, "*Alakh niranjan.*" These are the yogis who are teaching many people today, and they don't have even a little understanding of the truth. They think that you just wake up your kundalini and you become enlightened. Parshvanath never taught that you can become enlightened through kundalini awakening alone, just that you can make your body fully pure through working on your kundalini. With a pure body then you are ready to go deep into sadhana and find out what you really are. It takes a lot of effort. God appears in the pure thing, like a child. Even if you're 50 years old you become childlike, very innocent and pure. That divinity and purity is lost in the modern yoga tradition. *Alakh* means invisible, and *niranjan* means there is no dust or clouds around it. I means if you want to achieve the highest state of consciousness, you have to understand it is alakh niranjan; totally clear and pure. This is how Parshvanath described it. "Nath" means the lord, or owner, of oneself, and it started from Adinath. Samana and Shramana are other words for nath sect, but that is the true system, not the nath that's popular today. Many Tirthankaras were given the name with "nath," up to Parshvanath – he was the last one. These modern yogis have nothing to do with spirituality of the real nath system that started from the monks and nuns of the Tirthankaras. These new yogis are something special. They are fully polluted. They can call themselves *Siddha*, too. The misunderstanding i many people call someone who has achieved the siddhis, a Siddha. They can perform some kind of siddhi, or miracle, and people get easily trapped into it. It shows their ignorance, because Siddha is a liberated soul; they don't have a body anymore. Maybe these new yogis are just playing tricks, you never know. Like *Sathya Sai Baba*. People also called him Siddha Baba. Do you know what "sathya" means? It means "truth." He would manifest many things in front of people, like gold, little statues and ashes. He was just fooling them by performing illusion tricks. Everywhere it's known nowadays, but people are ignorant and still call him that.

You have to be very careful whom you are looking to for spiritual teachings. Never get trapped into the *"akhada* system." The akhada ashrams are where *Naga-Babas* live. Naga means "naked." Their lives are very strange, and they're corrupted because of money. These sadhus do a lot of things not acceptable in society. These sects call themselves sadhus and yogis, yet they drink alcohol or use drugs and smoke; some are even given the title of *Maha Mandle-Swaras*, the great, great swami. They're not supposed to sleep on beds or use furniture, according to their own way. It's a very difficult system if they follow it, but it became corrupted after Parshvanath. Hundreds of sadhus will live together and they get into really bad fights. Sometimes they go so far as to kill each other. And they're called yogis? A real yogi expands his consciousness and feels as if everything is a part of him or herself. They are nonviolent people. If these sadhus want to be the first to bathe in the Ganges River, they will fight each other and on some occasions innocent people have been killed by them, just so they can go in the river before anybody else. And people are bowing to these so-called yogis? The Ganges is not your own river. You can bathe first or bathe last, what is the big deal? Stay away from these kind of ashrams. They put ashes all over their bodies and they're very dirty people. The tradition is coming from the same place, but it became totally polluted when it branched off. These yogis, swamis and sadhus live in established ashrams and politics begin to enter because of the money. Spirituality totally disappears from these places. They are not really working to improve themselves and only want to have power and followers.

It's unfortunate that many people travel to India and get stuck following these sadhus. In Haridwar and Rishikesh they're always smoking *sulpha*, marijuana, even out in the open for everyone to see. Police won't even try to arrest them because they respect them. They mislead many people in the name of the Gita or other holy books and people are mesmerized by books like those because they're so old. Antique things become so popular. They don't have right vision, so they interpret them in their own way and spread the wrong messages. They're corrupted by money in a lot of cases. Be careful of these swamis. There are good swamis, but not in the majority. Here and there you can find a good swami, but they are unknown in public. Most of the swamis are into drugs, especially the well-known swamis. They become like kings because people think they are a kind of god and their ego goes so high.

If someone learns yoga these days everyone calls them a yogi. Yogi doesn't mean you learn some postures. It means the person is on the right path and working through all the steps to remove their ignorance. You don't call yourself a yogi; it is just what you become along the way. Yogis in India don't reach the highest state of consciousness.

People are so mesmerized when they see someone who can move their body in strange ways and suck their stomachs in very far, because a common person can't do it. They assume there is something special about them. It doesn't mean anything. Inside, their life is not that good, but people are people and get mesmerized by tiny things. Even Western people were so attracted to Sathya Sai Baba, because he said he could manifest things out of thin air. Nobody can do that. He told his followers the age he would die and he actually died four years prior to the date he gave. When he did die, they opened his room and found millions of dollars

– hundreds of kilos of gold. What would he do with all that money? He's a baba? A saint? People are too ignorant. He could have opened many hospitals or schools in poor areas all over the world. He had diamonds and jewelry, and so much gold and silver. All of it was in his room. He never allowed anyone to enter his room and he kept the key with him all the time. When he died, did all of the gold go with him? Even today Westerners are still fond of him and they even know the truth.

Stay away from people like this. If they're teaching you something good and not playing tricks, then maybe you can learn something. The majority of sadhus are not real. Many yogis are not real yogis. Many Babas are fake Babas. There are good among them, but they're not known, because the corrupted ones spoiled the name for the good ones. They stay out of politics and bad situations, so no one knows who they are.

Yoga is supposed to make you fully pure. In India the yogic system is well-known, and it comes from the Sanskrit root "*yujir yoge,*" which means "reunite with God." Many of today's scholars who have studied yoga have missed the point. They never mention the original center. The navel is the main center of the body, and all yogic practices are related to this center. Have you ever seen a baby sleeping? If you observe them quietly, you'll notice that the baby is breathing from the navel. That is why babies are so charming and beautiful to everyone. Why are you not equally attractive? Have you thought about it? Maybe you get up early to take a shower and use many lotions and other things. A lot of time is spent trying to improve your appearance every day, but you are still not as attractive as a butterfly, flower, plant or an animal. They don't wear makeup to cover their blemishes, but still they are very beautiful, very charming. The whole of nature is beautiful. Why is nature so beautiful? The answer is very simple: natural creatures live as they were born. They have not changed, they have not disconnected themselves from their origin. A baby is still connected with their origin, still breathing from the navel, and every baby is attractive, regardless of race, because they are as they were born. You become sick and unhappy because you start breathing from the chest. Thus you have cut off your connection from your center, the center of love. It's not your fault; the fault of ignorance is from generations and generations.

There is a story from India about a child who made a mistake, so his father slapped him. The child was surprised, and after a moment he asked his father, "Daddy, did your father slap you, too?"

"Yes!" said his father.

"Did your father's father slap him, too?" the boy asked.

"Yes, he did. Why are you asking such silly questions?" The father was becoming angry. The child said,

"Daddy, I will keep asking until I get to the bottom of this nonsense, because I want it to stop right now."

The child is right. You should immediately stop absurd or silly activities. Think about who you were as a baby, how beautiful and attractive you were. You loved everything. You were not afraid of even a snake or a lion, because you were pure and natural in your infancy. You were not concerned, worried, or afraid. A baby never thinks, "This is bad," or, "This is good." They see goodness and beauty everywhere. They love everything and only know beauty and love. No wonder nobody is afraid of a baby. They are still connected to their center. So, be like a child, be pure-hearted.

The 24th Tirthankara Mahavira said, "*Dhammo sudhassa chitthai.*" It means that the path can only exist in a pure heart. It's very important. If you want to develop your soul and realize God, or to know about the mysteries of life and death, then you have to start from the beginning. You must have a pure heart like a baby, because only you can follow your soul.

You are the greatest soul, the *paramatma*. The only difference is that you're diluted; you are partial paramatma, because there are illusions and attachments mixed up in you. Paramatma is like water. It can be a bucket of water that's dirty and full of trash, or it can be more clear like water from a clean river. This is *mahatma*, the great soul. Or, it can be perfectly clear water from the cleanest rainfall; this is *paramatma*, the pure soul. Water is water. We just use the different words to describe whether the water is more pure or less pure. Or, you can say that paramatma is like the sky on a perfectly clear and sunny day, but you are the sky with many clouds and a chance of rain. Still the sunshine is the same, there are just things in the way. The reason for the difference is that you do not always follow your heart completely. You only follow it partially, and only sometimes. As we grow up we lose touch with our center, and we need to find it again so that the path can be in our hearts.

Notice how animals treat their babies, it's very natural. Or, how many poor families or less educated people treat them. It is beautiful. At a bus station or airport you can observe many different people. The well-dressed, professional people are sitting up straight, their children are sitting in a separate chair, stiff and bored. "Be quiet, sit up straight, don't slump, don't fidget, you can play when we get home," is what you might hear from their parents. But the children of the poorer families are on their mother's laps or sitting on the floor playing with her feet, or standing on the chair behind her leaning over her shoulder, and she is petting them and singing to them. The big children are sitting on the floor cuddling their little brothers and sisters. Some of them may be playing a little game. They are happy, they are loving each other, and they don't care how long they have to wait for the bus. It's because they are being more natural than the other children who are always worried of upsetting their parents. Before a baby learns to walk, they have already become diplomatic in their actions. They smile and make gestures not to express their real feelings, but to fulfill the expectations of the parents, or to evoke something from them. There is one psychologist, an American named William James, and paraphrasing his words, he said that we think we frown because we are sad, or that we smile because we are happy, but really it is just the opposite. It's because we smile that we are happy.

Happiness is just the sensation of a smile as it feels from inside of us, plus the sensation of the heart and breathing in a healthy state – a state of relaxation. So, for an innocent baby, a sensation starts at the heart and their breath, then the smile follows, and the whole combination is felt as happiness – innocent happiness. But they learn quickly to make a smile and manipulate their body language, and their smiles start from the lips, no longer the heart. Then all the coordination of their body becomes confused. The lips are smiling, but the breath is tense. A smile that starts from the lips destroys the harmony of the whole body and the emotional system. When someone's facial expressions and gestures begin following someone else's actions instead of one's own natural rhythm, it becomes impossible to experience true emotions. The person has a lot of confusion and frustration inside of them, or simply shuts off their own awareness to avoid the conflict. This is how we became separate from our centers. The consciousness moves gradually away and upward to the mind. It's a matter of where we pay attention to in our bodies. Whatever sensations we choose to focus on when our attention is free, that is also where all of our movements will start from. A baby, an animal or a person deep in meditation lets their attention rest in the movement of the breath in the abdomen, near the navel. This is always a very relaxing and pleasant sensation. The rhythm of this area cannot be affected by someone else. When a young person is learning to behave, or become civilized, they focus their attention on their belly and chest. This is an area of feelings, but they can be controlled by other people in response to praise and criticism. The actions are controlled in the chest as the child worries about spilling their milk, or crying, because it will upset their parents. As they mature further, the center of attention rises up to the throat and they begin to think in words. They aren't spoken out loud, but the throat, tongue and chest create the motions that they would if they were speaking out loud. In the throat center, the actions are controlled by words; "I have to do this, I have to do that," and so on. When we think like this all the time, it means we're living in the throat. That is our center if our attention is there. We imagine what the outcome will be if we say a certain phrase to someone, maybe to a possible new boss in an interview. When we are in the throat all the time, we are aware of how to manipulate others with our own words, and we often put blame on others, make excuses, beg and plead for what we want. Finally the attention moves to the mind and to patterns of tension in the muscles, face and scalp. Whenever a person is frowning or grimacing, they are thinking. Their face muscles make patterns of tension that help them to imagine things. By watching someone's facial expressions people can tell what they are thinking. When someone is centered in this kind of thinking and movements, it's very easy for others to affect them. Consciousness in this area is used to remember the variety of isolated facts and data that's necessary for getting along in the society – phone numbers, addresses and so on. Without living in the brain, it's difficult to be civilized or respected by the society. People feel that appropriate behavior will lead them to success and prestige, and they won't be like the poor families at the bus station. People are disturbed because they live in the head, alongside all of their thoughts. Once I read about a man who put a name plate on his door with three degrees: "B.S., M.S., and Ph. D." His coworkers were surprised and asked him where he got all of his degrees, because they didn't know he went to college even.

He said to his coworkers, "Do you know what these stand for? B.S. – Well, you already know what that means. M.S. means more of the same, and Ph. D means, 'Piled high and deep.'"

All such knowledge belongs to the head. It is not necessary for you to have it in your mind if you want to live in your center. But education is important to get through the society, so I always recommend for people to complete their education. Learning never stops. For your whole life you will continue learning more and more. It's better to live in the heart than the head. Your heart is very close to soul itself. You can become paramatma if you are on the right track. If you start from the heart, you will reach to your soul one day.

It is good that you disconnected from your center. Everybody has to temporarily be cut off from their center if they really want to develop themselves, because until you learn things and collect a lot of knowledge, you will not have the chance to see through them to the reality. You can experience for yourself the futility of things. No matter how many things you collect, you will always find problems and insecurities.

In one story, there was a king who was hunting in the forest. After some time he left the path and realized he was lost. The sun was shining hard and he became too hot from carrying the weight of all of his gold jewelry, and was on the verge of having a heat stroke. He looked everywhere but could find no water at all. Suddenly he came across a naked man who lived in the forest. The king begged him for some water even begging with folded hands to this person he thought was a savage. He told him that he would give all of his diamonds and jewels for one drink of water. But there wasn't any. The naked man replied that there is no water, none at all. Think about it. If the king had all the money available to him and was hunting in his own kingdom, it shows that all of that money could not even satisfy his thirst. If there is no water, his money is useless. I suggest to people to understand the true nature of things and not be proud of possessions or their accumulation of knowledge. You can't take it with you. When you die, none of it can come with you. Nobody will be able to help you when death comes. Only if you find out the truth of what you are, that you are soul, only then can you die in peace.

It's a good thing that you got cut off, because now you can reunite with your center and develop yourself very quickly. Take for example a plant. If you cut off one branch, you can graft it back on. Normally, this is done when a farmer wants to put a branch on a different tree, but even when you graft it back where it came from, the same result happens. The branch is connected again, but this time it is not the same. It is much better. It will give better flowers, more foliage, and will produce better fruits than it did originally. The same thing applies to you after you've been disconnected from your center. When you reunite you will be unique. Come back to your home. Your real home is your center, your soul, your heart. Why are you running here and there? Why are you roaming around in your head? Remember the old proverb, "East or West, home is best." If you're in the head or chest, your mind is wandering in the East or the West. It is better to come back to your home, to your soul. Turn back and find where you started from.

When an individual begins to feel oneness with other creatures in their own heart, they will begin to adopt an attitude of living without harming or hurting anything. You'll understand that whatever you don't like, what causes you pain and discomfort, other creatures also feel the same. This person will forget all the theories they've been taught, which say that other creatures are the enemies of man. When you look at a snake or an insect and think, "They have the same feelings I do; what do they really want?" then you will not feel afraid anymore. You will not think that you have to kill it, or that it wants to hurt you. It is just living, the same as you are, but you happened to come across each other. It doesn't mean the insect or the snake is trying to hurt you just because you see them. There are very few problems when you feel this oneness. You think, "Why is this creature in this location? How does he feel, what does he want?" When you think like this, you see there is really no problem. If there is a fly in your house, maybe it's there to eat some food that you spilled on the countertop. When you clean up the food and it will have nothing to eat, and will go away. You needed to clean the kitchen sooner or later, so just do it and the fly will leave. There's no problem. If a bee is inside and bumping against the glass of a window, if you think about it, you will realize the bee just wants to go outside. So you can help them then. It's simple. 99% of the time, all creatures are helping each other to survive. Even a small ant or lizard is not useless on this earth. Remember that you are here, living on this planet, because of the cooperation of other living beings, other creatures. Animals depend on humans; humans depend on animals. If there were no flies, mosquitos, bees or butterflies, trees would give no fruit. Plants could not blossom flowers, and vegetables and grains would not grow without the insects to pollinate them. Even the snake has an important role many don't know about. In India, there is a word for snake, which is, "*pavanahari*." It means "the one who swallows the air." The snakes eat particles that float in the air, thus purifying the air and cleaning it. You can imagine that snakes are full of poison because they've swallowed all of the poisonous particles out of the air; that might help you to see they are not an enemy. It is just a way to think about it.

Return back to your center and reconnect yourself. Feel oneness with all creatures, all living beings on the planet. Everyone is beautiful here. Nature has given birth to all of us. All creatures are brothers and sisters, and all are children of nature, so don't harm them. We all depend on each other. When you understand what nature is, why nature gives birth to us, then you will feel love and oneness with other creatures. Then you will automatically be on the right track. Your energy will begin to flow upward and you will have the opportunity to become spiritual. This is what yoga is supposed to do in your life, but you have to follow all the steps. If you skip them because you're not interested, then whatever you're doing has nothing to do with yoga at all. You will be far from the spiritual path, and even further from lighting your soul.

SPIRITUAL TRADITIONS OF INDIA

The word "Hindu" is not a very old word. It used to be Sindhu before, but after some time the "S" was dropped, so they started calling them Hindu. Like Jain, it's also not a very old word. It started about 150 years after Mahavira. Before they were called many names through time such as *Samanopasak*, Samana, Shramana, Tapas, or *Jinopasak:* devotees of the Jinas, enlightened ones. The system is the oldest, but there was no word "Jain" until after Mahavira. Same thing with Hindu, but the word itself is just a little older than the Jain word. It was how we used to call the people. There was no religion known as Hindu. It meant whoever lived south from the Sindhu River, all the way to the ocean. If you lived there you were a Sindhu, or Hindu. No matter what system of teachings they were following everyone was known there as that. The people who live in India we call Indian. No matter which religion they follow we call them Indian, right? In America, you're called an American, no matter if you're Christian, Catholic, Buddhist or anything else. Same way, everyone was known as a Hindu. It means they lived in Hindu land – the Indus Valley.

Even though all the religions are separate, Hinduism represents all of them. What happened lately is that people began to forget the real sadhana, the real spiritual path of enlightenment, and they practice more rituals. It's because with the rituals they claim they will get quick results; if you're poor, do a ritual and you'll become rich suddenly; if you can't have a child, do a ritual and you'll be able to have a child. There's a *pooja*, or ritual, for everything. There were many beliefs like this and people just got trapped in it over time. The majority of people forgot the path of awakening the soul, burning the karma and liberating the soul. Some people tried to keep the system but through so many years people are interested more in getting money, a family, respect and status, these kinds of things, and the ones who had carried the true spiritual teachings died.

In Mahavira's time it was even worse. They began sacrificing animals by the name of religion in fire ceremonies. Not only that, they were doing the same with human babies. That was the worst period – Mahavira and Buddha's time. No wonder people began to follow the real system again that time. People practice and want to change when they are in suffering. It went too far and too extreme those days, so the people began to break those backward ideas and learn spirituality again from Mahavira.

All the religions in the Hindu culture wanted quicker results. They began worshipping angels more; we call them *devas*. It is a misconception that Hinduism is full of millions of gods. The truth is that it is full of angels. These angels live on their own planets and have very long lives. People pray and ask them for help in education, protection and safety, fame, love, things like this. It keeps them interested in it and they feel like someone is helping them, so these kind of prayers took over the real practice. Angels are worshipped even more than God in Hindu culture, which they believe God is one. It's unfortunate that most Hindus are not seeking enlightenment, but instead are seeking only the grace of God for everything to happen in their lives. They're not bad people, but they're keeping themselves away from enlightenment with these ideas. They ask

God for everything, blame God for everything and praise God for everything, never taking responsibility or putting effort to work for something in their life.

There are many religions within Hinduism, and many illusions. There is a path of Krishna's teaching which is widely known: *Radha* and *Krishna*. Even though Radha was not his wife, they worship them both together. In childhood, Krishna and Radha were friends. They spent some time together, and when he was 12, Krishna left that town. They never met again, not once. It's symbolic, if you read deeply in Krishna's teachings in the Gita or whatever else is available, you might find that Radha is a special thing. Radha is the path, and Krishna is absolute – pure consciousness. How do you reach that highest consciousness? They teach you in India you have to say, "*Radhe, Radhe, Radhe, shyam se mila de.*" The path is very difficult. You have to become like Radha. It means if you reverse *dhara*, it becomes radha. It's current, energy and force, and can bring you on to the path. You have to be very strong to do sadhana. The path can take you towards enlightenment if you reverse your dhara to radha, and that's the way you reach to krishna. "Krishna" means "consciousness," it's not a name in the real sense, but Hindus changed it fully and lost the real meaning in it. Krishna was a real person, that's sure, but not like what Hindus think of him. He was actually the cousin of the 22nd Tirthankara, *Neminath*, and they were very close friends. To make your energy reach to krishna, absolute consciousness, you need a tremendous current. Many ignorant Hindu sects tell you that if you just say the names of Radha and Krishna you will go higher upward. That is their ignorance. Radha is the name of the path. If they can teach that, then they will reach the highest state one day by following the system. Dhara needs to be Radha. If Radha never was able to meet Krishna after he left, how do you think she will take you to meet him? The truth is very difficult to hear, difficult to digest fully, and even more difficult to follow it. It is not that you know the truth; no, it is very difficult to digest. How will you know it? A little truth is even difficult to understand, and no one wants to see it.

There is a saying in India, "*Door ke dhol suhawane.*" If somebody is beating the drums from far away, they sound so beautiful, but if someone beats the drums close to you, it bothers and annoys you. It's a true saying. Sadhus and swamis will just put the three big stripes across their forehead, make a fire and everyone thinks they're good Babas, holy people. Do you know what they do at night? *Charas bhang, sulpha*; they smoke marijuana. That's what they do all night. Because if they're sitting out in cold weather, totally naked, they will die. They are drug-addicted, most of them. A few swamis I've met were good, but mostly not. They don't know the path; they depend only on Krishna. They are thinking, "It's very difficult to approach Krishna. Who can make the approach for me? Radha." They keep repeating all day, "*Radhe, Radhe, Radhe...*" As soon as Krishna left from Gokul she was never able to see him again. He went to south India. If she couldn't meet him herself how will she take you there? Still they dance around singing this all the time. Hindus say through Radha, Christians say through Jesus. That's the way they do things – without effort. Meet God yourself. What's wrong with you that you can't do it? You can meet it if you put the right efforts. Learn good things, do your sadhana. You don't need something to take you. Just go.

It's difficult because swamis don't have a history of their own lineage. Where they come from, maybe they think only seven lines or a hundred maximum, but not any further. They just add whoever is popular to their lineage. I mentioned earlier that when Adinath gave himself diksha, initiation onto the spiritual path, many kings, queens, princes and princesses renounced and followed him as a monk or nun. He didn't receive food for a year because they were giving him jewelry or gifts when he went to a home, and a Tirthankara never speaks for food. The monks and nuns started leaving him. They were starving and went back to society wearing colored clothing. "These clothes indicate we are weak," they told people if they were asked why they left the Tirthankara. Colorful clothes in those days, made with natural dyes from soil and so on, indicated that you were emotionally weak. That's the way all the different sects started, when they left the path and branched off.

In the beginning they were still okay though, they were following the best they could. The most popular swami sect was started by Adinath's grandson, Maarichi, who became Mahavira 24 lives later. He never made a disciple in his whole life; he would send everyone to Adinath and tell them he is the real thing. He knew he didn't know the truth himself, so he inspired thousands and thousands of monks and nuns, and that collected the karma to become a Tirthankara. Later, people might have said they were his disciples because they used to live around him, but he never initiated anyone. I can give an example: suppose that today someone claims to be a disciple of Yogananda. They are claiming that way, but maybe they met him for just one day, or maybe they never met him and only follow his teachings. Maybe Yogananda was not even enlightened. An enlightened master would never write an autobiography. Maarichi never initiated a single disciple, but people claimed they were his disciples, and that's how swami sects began. There is actually no such thing as a Hindu swami. It makes more sense to say an Indian swami. These swamis who consider it Hinduism don't have the right history, and it's not their fault either.

The real history was burned in the 8th century. It was preserved in the Buddhist monasteries; all the history of India was there. In those monasteries, Adi Shamkaracharya was so powerful in logic that he defeated all the Buddhists. Buddhists enjoyed debating and after he defeated them with his arguments he ordered for every one of their monasteries to be burned to the ground. All the literature of India was in those monasteries because King Ashoka put it there. Thousands of monks and nuns were in those monasteries; can you believe how big the libraries could have been? The real history is gone, because he wanted to recreate his own history. Adi Shaṁkaracharya must have been a very egotistical person. Modern people believe he was a god. Having defeated the Buddhists in the debates, all the history is gone forever. Buddhists will never forgive him. Even though later in his life he became more humble, down to earth and changed himself a lot, they will never forgive him. You're not supposed to burn your own country's history. That's wrong to do. Jain teachings weren't lost, because they didn't keep them in one place; they were with the monks and nuns wherever they went. Adi Shaṁkaracharya debated with Jains, too, but he wasn't able to defeat any of them.

The difference between the monks and nuns of the Samanic system and the tradition of swamis is that swamis are flexible; they are not complete followers of nonviolence, most of them. I was invited to a Hindu temple in America by a swami there and talked with him after speaking with the people. I asked his name and he was telling me about the president of the temple. I said that he must be vegetarian, and I was shocked at his reply. He said there is no need to be a vegetarian because his devotion is enough. The ignorant Hindus like this think whatever they do in their life, God will forgive them for it. Do bad things every single day and then pray to God – you'll be forgiven. Then it means you can go and kill people and pray to God afterwards. That kind of ignorance is what swamis carry. They are not following the path of spirituality and sadhana, the real path of nonviolence. They consider themselves spiritual teachers;

they should be teaching that vegetarian is the first step to becoming nonviolent if they really want to be a spiritual teacher. They think if a person is a meat-eater, but they are very devoted to God, then it's okay; God will forgive them. That is the difference between swamis and monks and nuns of the spiritual path. Monks will never compromise with violence, not once. No matter what situation, they will not eat meat or cause harm. Maybe they are not very wise monks if they get in the situation where there is no food available for them to sustain their body except for meat, but they still would rather die. That is the discipline swamis are lacking. It's because they don't have the right teachings; all of the branches that split away in the past started doing their own things, and they forgot the science of how karma works and practicing real sadhana for the soul.

In the very beginning the swamis were still okay. They were still close in time to Adinath and had other Tirthankaras in the future, but after splitting so many times and making more and more separate sects they forgot the reality and began teaching how they interpreted things. They told people to just sit with a fire all the way around you and it's a big austerity, like Kamatha was performing when Parshvanath saw him. Things like that went far away from true sadhana and made them egoistic. They continued to mislead people for their hunger of respect. At least Kamatha was an ascetic; he lived with a lot of discipline but unfortunately mislead people.

The Brahmanic tradition was at the beginning, too. The Brahmans were like Samanas, having renounced, but they went the wrong way just like the swamis did. They were doing sadhana and had some discipline, but they began to consult householders and give predictions about their life, promise that things would get better, to not worry about this or that, it will all get better. Monks are not supposed to be involved in these things, because you never know, what if they tell someone it will get better and then their family member dies? So, they went off the path and started doing rituals for the people, telling them it would help with their problems. In those days rituals were just a few minutes, not hours and hours like they are today. There was not much difference, but later on it became a big gap when they went away from the Samanic system.

In the beginning of Jainism, as a religion, approximately 2,400 years ago, there were no rituals. At that time they were still focused merely on awakening the soul and indulging in their sadhana. No matter if they belonged to the Digambara or Shvetambara sect. They wanted only right understanding. It happened closer to the 8th century that rituals came in and the monks started losing the right concepts. When Hinduism was reestablished, belief in the incarnation of Vishnu became popular. For Jains, there was no dancing, no singing; in dancing you kill living beings, and in singing you kill living beings. Therefore, Jain spiritualism seemed like a dry path. This is where the *Acharyas*, the leaders of monks and nuns, started getting stuck into extreme disciplines without understanding the meaning. On the other hand, *Vaishnavas*, devotees of Vishnu, were dancing, singing, beating drums; it was beautiful and people began to join in. Jain Acharyas thought the people would become Vaishnavas instead of Jain, so they started to write new books and included some fire ceremony rituals and *aartis*, devotional songs, in order to attract and convert people to Jainism.

This is the time when Jainism lost its spiritual depth and they wanted more people to be Jain. They started trying to convert people more than practice their own sadhana. Before this happened they weren't worried about it. If people wanted to learn and practice sadhana that was okay, and if they didn't, it didn't bother them. They were always deep in their spiritual practices and meditation, working to improve themselves. Rituals came into Jainism in this way, but mostly they are practiced by the Digambara sect.

Nowadays, all of these Jain monks and nuns, especially in Gujurat and Rajasthan, they got stuck into *kriyas*. It means a kind of action; don't touch this water, don't touch this dirt, don't eat that, don't eat this. It's the daily routine, how to do things and conduct their lives. When they go to collect alms, there are 42 rules to go by, and they stick with them strictly. They think if they follow these 42 rules they are burning their karma. They got too absorbed and stuck into those rules instead of doing the right thing. All the Tirthankaras were sitting in lotus posture at some time. How many Jain monks or nuns know yoga? If you go to India today, most of them are sick because they eat the best food, the richest food. They don't even know they are eating that food because they don't have sense to think about their bodies anymore. Even though the body is the instrument for the soul, they don't think about it. Most Jains are wealthy and they want to give monks and nuns the best food. The monks go to the Jain houses now, the same houses every day, where they receive rich food that's full of cholesterol. Everything is cooked in *ghee,* clarified butter, and very greasy. It's not good food to eat. The system the Jain monks follow says that you only go to collect food at houses that are unfamiliar to you. This way you become very humble. Maybe the house you go to for food one day doesn't appreciate monks and they say harsh words to you, or tell you that you're wasting your life by being a monk. At the same time, you aren't dependent on the same family for food, and cause them a burden by going day after day. This is the way monks and nuns are supposed to go for food, but they don't even follow that anymore.

Monks are supposed to be free. The ascetic path means freedom, but in India they live in so much fear. Every day they go to the same house, and most of the time householders will take them around so they don't have to find the houses themselves. Jains are giving their spiritual teachers unhealthy food all the time. If you eat like that, at least do yoga so your body becomes healthier and you can digest it. They do kayotsarga for only two minutes, maybe. Two minutes won't do anything. Routine and rules have taken over their path and they don't even put much effort to improve themselves. They memorize their *pratikraman*, a kind of confessional verse, but they don't even say it with their heart if they made a mistake during the day. They just memorize it and repeat it every day, morning and evening. If they stepped on a bug while they were out walking that day they will just say the pratikraman three times. It's like a routine for them – not in their hearts at all. The words are mechanical and have no meaning. They're stuck, but it's not their fault. They just don't understand history and how the changes over time have affected them. The last Tirthankara, Mahavira, did a lot of kriyas like this. Because he had more karma than all of the previous 23 Tirthankaras combined, he had to go through them and burn them the hard way. The monks and nuns began to follow him, imitate him. Tirthankaras say not to imitate them because they are doing what their body can tolerate, and for their own specific karmas. Maybe you can learn a lot of discipline from imitating them, but they did it for the reason of burning their remaining karma. Since the writing system really began just after Mahavira's time, they collected all of his teachings that had been memorized by many people still living, so, all of these Jain scriptures that are available come mostly from those teachings and are full of rules, because of the Shramanas imitating the way he was living.

Jains today think if you do pranayama (breathing exercises), you kill the living beings in the air and collect lots of karma. When you do yoga postures and move your body and limbs you also kill all the living beings in the air. Yes, there are living beings all around in the air, but they don't know the truth that this type of living being is so flexible, they can adapt. We inhale, exhale, inhale, exhale all of these bacteria since the first day we're alive. It's a natural process, and the natural things won't block you from reaching enlightenment. Mahavira taught to minimize the violence, even though your mere existence means violence. Your body has to breathe in oxygen to be alive, so how will you do sadhana and work on yourself if you stop breathing? Same thing with the living beings in water. It's a lack of knowledge that the Jain monks and nuns have and they don't want to go through the understanding.

There are living beings everywhere, but it doesn't mean by breathing you will kill them all. You have to inhale and exhale. They are not in a conscious state anyway. In each moment, they are being born and dying thousands of thousands of times. They have only one sense, but they are not conscious so they don't feel anything. Their lives are so short they wouldn't have time to realize what they're feeling, anyway. In every moment they're born and they die at the same time. By the time you inhale one breath, they die and are born again many times before you even exhale. Even if you weren't breathing them in, they would be dying and being born in the same way just in the air alone. That's the state their soul is in: continuously in birth and death, unconscious. Jains are wrong not to do yoga and pranayama because of that fear. That's why I put all of these traditional Jain monks and nuns down since the very beginning.

Because of their fear to break traditions, the universal principles are not spread all over. They are scared to go on a ship because the ship will kill the living beings in the water. They don't understand the state that those living beings are in; they don't have that knowledge. They are not the only ones using the ship. If they go or don't go, the ship will still go with other people. You have to do some things that are necessary, otherwise the truth will be stuck in a tiny place for a few people. The teachings are supposed to be available everywhere, for everyone. They have to get out of this dilemma. Ashoka, the great king, asked the Acharyas to send their monks and nuns everywhere to spread the teachings, but those Acharyas were so ignorant they didn't accept his idea. They didn't want to travel because when you walk from place to place you kill living beings. Ashoka's second choice was the Buddhist teachings, and they accepted his idea. The Buddhists broke their tradition, so now Buddhism is everywhere because of them. It became so popular and there is not even much truth left in it anymore.

Tirthankaras don't make sects or convert people. If someone comes to them and asks a question, they will tell them what they need to hear in order to wake up their soul. Mostly Catholics come here to Siddhayatan, and they enjoy learning. Why? Because we don't try to convert them. Whatever path somebody else is on, it has nothing to do with your soul, it makes no difference to you. But people get the idea stuck in their minds that they have to make other people share their ideas.

We need spiritual vision to help us grow. These teachings were locked in India because of the ignorance of those Jains. The householders are not less ignorant than the monks and nuns. Still today, they resist and condemn those who leave India such as myself. They think if you ride in the car or airplane that you are killing so many living beings; therefore, you're not the real monk. You cannot share the teachings with anyone if you refuse to travel. Their own scriptures tell them that they will have to adjust their lifestyle according to the time and place in which they live. It doesn't mean you compromise the principles, only that you make changes in your traditions that don't work anymore. They think that giving food to a monk is collecting the biggest virtue; they think they did the best job in the world. What about their other needs? They don't even ask. In many areas of India they will ask the monks and nuns if they need toothpaste or other items. In Gujurat, a state of India, if a monk uses toothpaste they will say they're not a good monk. The monks are considered "good" if they're dirty. If their clothes are dirty, they will come to you even more. It's called the "ornaments of the monk;" the dirtier and smellier the monk is, the better they are. Because of their backward ideas the real messages didn't spread. The whole world wants to learn yoga and meditation. The whole world is becoming aware of nonviolence and vegetarianism. The world is ready, but they don't want to even move from their place in India, because they have so many fears. The Jain monks and nuns are still the most resistant, yet they're the ones who should be teaching meditation and yoga postures, pranayama and spiritual principles.

The Jain word itself has a beautiful meaning. It comes from the word *Jina*, the one who has dissolved *raga* and *dwesha* – attachment and hatred. We call them Jina in the Prakrit language. Devotees of Jina are called Jain. When you dissolve raga and dwesha, it means you burn all the major karmas associated with them and you reach enlightenment. If you know how to write in Hindi, the two vowels above the "Ja," the two lines, indicate raga and dwesha. A Jain means one who is trying to win over raga and dwesha. If they will dissolve and win over them one day, they will become a Jina. Until then, they remain Jain. Anyone, any truth-seeker, can be a Jain.

Today Jains are maybe too much into traditions. They don't know the science because they're not scholars. I've met many professors of Jainism, and deep down they know that many of their traditions are not good, because they have studied a little bit of history about them. On the outside it appears as though they're doing good, but on the inside they know it doesn't matter. What matters is to do sadhana. Just like the Tirthankaras taught – to do fasting, meditation, yoga, mantras, and pranayama. Not everyone can fast. Out of 10,000 people, maybe one has a body that can handle fasting. There are many different kinds of bodies and many different paths. Jain scholars know how the traditions built up, but they live in the same traditions. You don't compromise the principles if they're right. The main principles are called *Mulaguna*. *Uttaraguna* are smaller things like rules, and these can change according to time. Everything changes according to time, but the Mulaguna are the deep principles that take you into your soul. Everyone is using cell phones, including the monks and nuns in India. They use Facebook and YouTube. The problem is that they hide it. They try to act innocent and say they don't know what it is, but they do know. If you can use technology as a tool to spread spiritual principles, then use it. If you're bright enough, you compromise the traditions according to time, then you can flourish.

Mahavira never taught religion or wished to establish one, and there was no word "Jain." Whenever you adopt a religion, it seems very good for you; there are good ideas in some religions. When I took diksha and was initiated as a Jain monk at 14, I thought the same way. However, as you begin to learn languages and can read all religious books, you begin to put together an idea of the reality of these religions, if you can see through it. Jains these days are lacking. They are too much into traditions that have no meaning today. How to go for food, how to wash or not wash yourself, how to drink water. In Mahavira's time there was no system of washing, or getting clean water to drink like today, so you had to do things a certain way in order to survive, but they're made according to that time. It doesn't make sense to do them today. I always differ from the traditions, but not the principles. *Pancha Mahavratta*, the five great-vows (nonviolence, truthfulness, non-stealing, celibacy and non-possession), was given by the Tirthankaras. They are universal principles and can be practiced by every person. You don't have to be a monk or nun to start. The best place to begin is where you are now.

PART II:
THE
CHAKRA SYSTEM

KUNDALINI

I'm often asked, "What is the kundalini energy? Why do they call it kundalini?" Yogis used to live in the Himalayas, and on their way through the mountains they encountered cobras, a very poisonous snake with a hood around its head. When the cobra rests, it coils its body and lays its head on top. It sleeps and rests, but if somebody teases it by throwing rocks, sticks or something else, the snake becomes so angry when its disturbed. It stands straight up in the air and looks around to see what disturbed it. A cobra is actually a very shy snake, but if it gets angry it will chase someone. So, yogis observed that when a cobra becomes angry its body became straight, from downward to upward, right away. Therefore, they gave the name kundalini energy, because our energy from the root chakra, *Muladhara*, all the way up to the crown chakra, *Sahasrara*, is supposed to be very active and flow upward. Like gaining all the energy and force to be transformed into radha, the path. If the energy is flowing downward the person will have sickness, feel heavy and lack mental clarity. Maybe they're mentally, physically or spiritually sick. The kundalini is where the energy flows. In Sanskrit, whoever coils their body is called *kundali*, and one who has kundali is called *kundalini*. Your energy needs to be active and alert like a cobra being woken up from its sleep. That's the kundalini energy, and it needs to flow from downward to upward through all the chakras.

There is a misconception about kundalini everywhere. First of all, the kundalini is not located in the base of the spine. It's located from the base of the spine all the way up to the top of the crown chakra; kundalini is the entire passageway. Kundalini is where your energy moves, and the seven chakras are from the base of your spine to the crown of your head. You have to make your energy very strong and forceful to move upward.

People want to know where the kundalini is coming from. Everyone is born with this energy and the chakras in their bodies. Without the energy we cannot even take birth in the human body; it won't be alive at all. Kundalini energy is just energy: life-force, chi, *prana*. Whatever name you choose to give to it, it is the energy in our bodies and it moves clockwise when it's healthy, in small areas just two inches in diameter. These areas are called chakras. It isn't made of anything because it has no structure. It's just energy, and you cannot touch it or grab it; it's not physical. Medically speaking, the energy is not visible, so it appears to not exist. However, the organs are there, so we can see how our energy is working by checking the health of our organs. That is one way.

We are all born with this energy, but not everyone has the same amount. Maybe someone's first chakra is partially blocked; they'll need to work on it a lot, since they have low vitality. Healthy chakras are supposed to spin clockwise, be strong and have a high current to move upward. That is called kundalini rising. Most people do not have healthy chakras.

Kundalini has a very important role in the human's life. If it flows properly in your body, flowing through the chakras in a balanced way, then you will be always healthy. It keeps you in good health, good mind and good thoughts. Maybe you think you are in good health now, but this is something different. When your energy is flowing properly through all your chakras it's difficult to imagine what your life would be like; you will never have a negative thought. You will be very compassionate, very loving, in every moment, even in sleep.

When kundalini is open and clear it means your *nadis* are clear and the breath flows in the center channel. You'll have chances to dive deep into meditation. Nadis are the main nerves in your body, your nervous system. Suddenly you will get in touch with your soul. It is something you can't imagine. When it really happens it's something special. The more balanced you are, the better hands you're in. Deep meditation will take you to your soul, and you need your kundalini to be very open to experience this. The chakras are cleared one by one as it moves all the way up to the seventh. They need to be active but not over-active. When your kundalini is moving too fast, you can have too much energy and end up into the wrong things. You might indulge in too much lust, either in your actions or thoughts, and the energy begins to flow down. Or, you might get stuck in feelings of hate, jealousy, violent thoughts, frustration, and all these lower emotions, thus causing your kundalini to flow down right away. It's instant.

Spiritual practices require a lot of energy. For example, maybe the first chakra is blocked and not creating energy, as a result there is no current, no dhara. It flows downward when there is no energy there, like a small stream flowing over the edge of some rocks. Naturally it will always go down. You need a tremendous current to change the direction. You need a dam to build up the energy. When the energy becomes an upward flow, that is when it becomes radha. If you want to reverse the flow of the downward energy, you need to make a big dam around it. It takes a lot of effort to make the dam. It's not an easy task. Same thing, the spiritual path is not easy. Radha is not easy. It's unfortunate that intelligent people like Osho didn't follow the system, otherwise they could have reached enlightenment. He said if you want to end your desire for sex, you have to have tremendous sex until you become allergic to it. That's what Osho was teaching. If you do that, you lose everything; there is nothing left in the body, all the energy is wasted completely. You will have no current, no force, no energy. It will never become radha if you follow the path of Osho. That's why I tell people you have to let your chakras be open and preserve your energy, make it stronger and it will flow upward. It's not easy to flow upwards, but somehow you have to do it if you are the spiritual person. The path of sex is not the way; you will lose everything.

Sex and spirituality is a hot topic, especially in the Western countries. They think by sex they can reach moksha, liberation, and become a liberated soul. In the East it is just the opposite; many cultures think sex is a bad thing. If you ask a Catholic priest, nun or monk, they say just to talk about sex is inappropriate. If you go to third world countries, like India suppose, there's a misconception about sex there, too. As soon as a teenager begins to ask questions about sex, it's called *gandibaat*, dirty talk. No one wants to talk about it. No wonder there are many rapes in this aspect, because they don't have knowledge about what sex is. I will criticize sex, because sex cannot take you to the higher level. Sex is a desire, a craving. That craving which is a hot topic in the Western countries today, they think they can enhance their energy by having sex and they're wrong.

In Sanskrit we call it "*kamvasana*." "Kam" means "sex," and "vasana" is the desire. Where there is a desire or craving for sex, your energy is going down and your chakras will never be awakened. People like Osho, they think sex takes you to enlightenment. They got trapped in it, even the whole organization. In Osho's ashram in India, you cannot even visit unless you are tested for the HIV/AIDS disease; it's required if you want to stay there. They have to have that test because Osho believed in open sex and the government is scared of AIDS spreading. Instead of going higher, they go downward. All Indian religions criticize sex, but not a single religion in India criticizes love. There are two things, there is desire and love. They always support love. They don't consider it sex. Maybe the act is the same, but it's a different meaning.

For sex, the Sanskrit word is "*manoj*" or "*manodbhav;*" it comes from your mind. Your mind creates this craving. Even if you don't have a partner, your mind will create the craving. That desire is dangerous, it becomes your addiction. As soon as you are in the desire of sex, your energy automatically goes down. And you want to be liberated? People are stuck in it and they're wrong. Instead of going higher their energy goes all the way down. They can never be spiritual if they continue.

When your kundalini has enough force to go from your first chakra (base of spine) to the second chakra (approximately 2 inches above the first), there can be a lot of sexual energy. The movement of energy in the second chakra creates the sexual energy. If the second chakra is clear, though, it will move up to the third chakra and you will be more balanced, less scattered.

It is not surprising that not a single person in the Western countries has ever been enlightened, even though many claim to be, because their concept is wrong. Maybe they're awakened, but not enlightened. They're too much into sex. Look at how sex dominates the media and entertainment industries. Energy needs to flow upwards through love and the positive qualities. Love is totally different from sex. If you have knowledge about how to be really moving into love, that love can create such an energy and aura around you that you can achieve the highest state of ecstasy. Ecstasy can be achieved through the proper way, but not by sex. Sex is a totally different act and needs to be criticized, but it doesn't mean you don't need to have knowledge. If you don't have knowledge it can be a dirty game. If you have knowledge it can be a blessing for you. Maybe you are married; if your partner and you flow in love, that love will create a beautiful aura around you and expand the love into your family, into your neighborhood, into your country. That's why we call it love, not sex. Sex needs to be criticized because it drains you. Love never drains you. Love always takes you higher.

Inquiries on the topic of sex are very good. You have to be more knowledgeable about it. It's not an easy subject, especially to understand the orgasm. Let me tell you. Freud is well known. Freud said, if you don't masturbate almost two or three times a day, you're not a human. It means he supported that idea. Osho also supported Freud. He promoted open sex in his commune. Osho's book is called *Sex to Superconsciousness*. First of all, you have to understand what the orgasm is. An orgasm happens when the soul gets an instrument. The body is an instrument for the soul. Why? Because soul is weak and weaker, the weakest, since centuries. It doesn't put effort to grow spiritually, to get enlightenment. The karmas are so thick around it, the clouds so dense. And all this other matter is so thick it's hard to see anything. So, the soul is blind, even though it knows everything. It gets this instrument, the human body, after a lot of improvement over millions of years. Animals have this instrument, but their instrument is not developed enough to realize who they really are, or what ecstasy and bliss are. The problem is that Westerners got stuck into sex and spirituality. They get attracted to it, and no wonder many people got trapped in Osho's commune and follow his teachings today. I often talk about sex, that sex is not our goal. Sex makes your energy flow down. The orgasm is a totally different thing. For example, the closest feeling to an orgasm is like when a person wakes early in the morning from sleeping and they have to go to the bathroom badly. With so much pressure and the release of urine, the body feels relaxed and very light. It's a kind of orgasm. But an orgasm is nothing; according to psychiatrists, an orgasm is just a releasing of energy when the muscles become very tense from stimulation, followed by endorphins being released throughout the body and it feels good. Like if your head is feeling congested and heavy and you suddenly sneeze, it's a little relief and you get a type of orgasm. It's a technique, and that technique is not taught in society. If that technique is taught, couples that are in love, can enhance their energy instead of wasting it. The technique was given in the ancient times of India, but they misused it. People forgot the real purpose of it. As long as they love each other, they have chances to enhance this energy up high. Basic energy is the sexual energy. According to Freud, masturbation releases the energy, but he didn't know it makes you weak. All the energy goes down and is wasted. It's a desire of sex. The Catholic priests are full of it, and they consider themselves celibate. Many of them masturbate secretly and don't even know how much energy they're losing. What happens if somebody does it with themselves and there is no other partner to give you the energy back? A male body is positive and a female body is negative – yin and yang we call it. So, the positive wires create the spark and enhance the energy, so neither of them loses energy. Because they're in love, they increase the energy more. The chances are when people are in love and flow in that love always, they don't lose the energy at all. Instead of losing, they gain it. When they are having merely sex, they use it and their energy goes down.

The orgasm in Sanskrit is "*brahmanandasahodara*," which translates as, "the brother of Brahma." Brahma is God. "Sahodara" means "brother." God is blissful, God is in ecstasy. Nature gives you the chance to experience the orgasm, if you know how to feel or realize it, so that you can understand that true bliss is more than that feeling. Even if you have some kind of relief, even if you feel very good, after releasing this energy with your partner, those feelings make you think that, is it coming from me or is it coming from the other? Ultimately, the two people who are in love, the orgasm happens within himself or herself. It doesn't come from the outside. It's an inner-phenomenon. Every time a person feels an orgasm, it is his own or her own. The other is just merely the cause to it, but if you learn the technique you can make it happen by yourself. You don't have to go through the sexual act or masturbation. There is also no desire for it. Suddenly, you are in deep meditation, and in deep meditation you have fully forgotten your body. You're suddenly thrown in that kind of bliss or ecstasy. You've never experienced it. You don't want to come back from there. Orgasm is nothing in comparison to this bliss.

Orgasm is like, suppose there are millions of layers of lights; the orgasm is like the first layer of the light, and bliss is like all the millions of layers of light. If you can experience all the millions of layers of the light at once, that is called bliss. There is no comparison to bliss. I always tell my students who make inquiries, don't be ignorant to have just one layer and miss millions of layers. Raise yourself so high that you can get those millions of layers, and you can see through it all at once. Can you imagine what bliss can be then? It is difficult to explain.

The people who are thinking they can go through the orgasm and grow spiritually are wrong. They can enhance their energy only if they are in love. They can help each other to grow, but the condition is that the other has to be on the same level. If one is on a higher level of spirituality and the other is fully low, it's not going to happen. The lower level person is going to suck your energy and there are chances they will both go down. That's why you have to consider, is your partner the same level? Do they have peace? Forgiveness? Kindness? A lot of patience and tolerance?

Let me explain, in another way, what an orgasm is or what bliss is. If you're a lady, sometimes you can have multiple orgasms. What is a multiple orgasm? It's the same idea. Multiple orgasms are like bliss. When they have multiple orgasms they have a little step ahead. It happens mostly in women's cases, and not as much in men's cases. Men are so aggressive, and they miss their opportunity. They don't know how to do it. If they drink, and after drinking they are having sex, they are not going to get anything, their energy will be released and they'll go down right away.

There are many interviews out there by "sex experts," and they say that if a girl drinks five or seven beers, she will be in heaven when she's having sex. They are wrong. She is under the influence of alcohol and the body is full of toxins. When the body is full of any toxins, you will not feel the real thing at all. That is killing your body's cells. The real people, when they want to enhance their energy, they need to be very pure. This instrument needs to be purified. For a man who wants to have multiple orgasms, he needs to learn the right breathing technique. They can go through multiple orgasms and it can give them a little idea that this is a little taste of what bliss can be. Unfortunately, most people get stuck and trapped into the orgasm, but don't want to improve spiritually to taste the real bliss.

The orgasm is a vacuum. In that state, when you are in climax, you don't have any thoughts, you don't have any mind, and that's what bliss is like. Bliss has no mind and no thoughts, but the orgasm is just a teeny-tiny taste. Don't compare this teeny-tiny taste with bliss. Bliss is still billions of miles away from you, but it shows that you have potential if you use this energy positively and wisely. Make your body pure. No toxins in the body. Make it fully light. If your partner is on the same spiritual level as you, then you can enhance your energies together and you both might be able to experience multiple orgasms. When you're moving in love, your whole consciousness, your whole soul is moving in love and it needs to open up. There is a way. I condemn those sexual activities but I am not against love. Love can enhance your energy.

You have to know the right technique from the yogic system. You also need to change how you eat. Purify this body, because this body can become divine. It's connected with God already, because we are part of God, we're not separate, but we lost this divinity already. When we lose this divinity we are going far away from the bliss. We are just in illusion to have these orgasms and these orgasms have no meaning.

I suggest that you never masturbate, especially if you want to balance your chakras. This is not called "self-love." Why? Because you don't gain anything at all. If you have a partner, that is different; you both gain when you are moving in love, not merely sex. So, no wonder many cultures condemn the sexual acts, but nobody condemns love. That's why sex and love are totally two different things. They are two different poles and you need to understand that. To summarize, the orgasm is a vacuum, and in that state thoughts disappear. In that state, when a person is in climax, moving in love, it will create that kind of vacuum and will bring you a little teeny-tiny taste of bliss. You can increase it to multiple orgasms, but you cannot increase it that way to go to bliss. Whoever is teaching you these wrong things, don't get trapped in that school or those teachings. Otherwise you will go downward and you will not be in that high state of bliss.

When you waste your energy through sex all your thoughts begin turning negative and taking you down. You feel depressed or apathetic. It takes a long time to bring your energy back up again. After your energy is wasted you have to make your thoughts pure and work on each of the lower three chakras. All of the energy leaves the second chakra down to the first and then is released. It will take a minimum of six months to create that energy reserve again through your sadhana.

By sex nobody has achieved liberation. Read the ancient techniques of India, the *Kama Sutra*. It explains how to enhance your energy if you have a good partner in love, but not one time does it mention sex. If it's real love, it can expand you, expand your soul. It will expand you on that level where all your chakras can be cleared out and your spirituality begins. Why is spirituality being seen by people as just another religion? Because they don't have the right knowledge about love. They got mixed up with sex. They're totally opposite poles. Choose one. If you want to go higher, choose love; if you want to go lower, choose sex.

Don't be confused about sex and spirituality. Where sex ends, spirituality begins. Only love prevails, and it means you are going upward. If you want to be a spiritual person, improve yourself and increase your energy instead of draining it. Awakening needs your increasing energy.

Sometimes people release sexual energy involuntarily while they're sleeping. This happens more or less because the body has extra energy that it can't use right away and it releases by itself. It doesn't affect a person's kundalini when this happens naturally. When it's released because the thought processes are involved in too many sexual thoughts, then that is a different story. If a person is really working on themselves and improving a lot through their spiritual practices, most of the time it will happen as a natural function of the body and has nothing to do with the sexual thoughts.

What about people who engage in sexual acts but do not release any of their energy? Firstly, only yogis can even do this, and very few yogis. These acts having nothing to do with sex when they do them the right way. Some yogis used to have a partner and be married, but not how we think of having a partner today. They used to enhance their energies, but never release it, and never indulge in sexuality or attraction. Maybe only a few yogis left nowadays are capable of those techniques, but it doesn't mean they are practicing them. When the yogis did those techniques they didn't have any lustful or negative thoughts involved in it; they did it for a different purpose. I don't recommend people to try these because it is very difficult, and can be dangerous.

When you are in any negativity, your energy flows all the way down right away. It's automatic, remember. As soon as the thoughts or emotions are in you, you go down. Any moment you have anger, your energy is flowing down. Anger doesn't mean you have to be yelling or fighting someone. What about when you are walking to your work and you spill your tea or coffee? That frustration comes from anger. Deceitfulness brings your energy down, too. Ego, jealousy, feeling possessive of something or someone, being greedy, working too many hours; all of these make your kundalini energy flow down and you'll never achieve bliss. What about eating meat, over-eating, drinking alcohol, using drugs or smoking? Not only do these make your energy flow down, but at the same time you are hurting your body. And you say you want to be spiritual and reach enlightenment? The purpose of kundalini is to make your body fully pure, healthy and clean, but you are wasting your time when you continue to pollute and damage your body with these things. Your kundalini practices, your chakra practices, yoga practices – none of your spiritual practices mean anything if you are doing any of these things. Go to a yoga studio and you can hear many people talk about awakening their kundalini and reciting "*aum shanti*," but the practices have no effect if one hour you sit and recite mantras, and the next hour you go to drink with your friends. It doesn't make sense. If you want to raise your kundalini you better drop these things. I appreciated Yogi Bhajan in this particular aspect. He was teaching people about vegetarianism, and his movement became very popular. Fifty-percent of Sikhs are not vegetarian, so if some of them were inspired by him then that's very good.

Yogi Bhajan, who is known for Kundalini Yoga, was not actually a yogi. He gave himself his own name, but he never did yoga practices. Even if someone is a real yogi, the word yogi is not part of their name. He taught his whole system and related it to the Sikh teachings, which are primarily found in northern parts of India. The Sikh book, *Guru Granth Sahib*, is a very beautiful book. It's a collection of Hindu, Jain and Buddhist teachings, and there are also a few yogic techniques that Yogi Bhajan found in it.

When he came to America to teach, it was good timing for him, because he noticed that many people were being drawn towards India and eastern teachings. He didn't teach the real kundalini system. When he taught, he related things to the *Guru Granth Sahib*, which is mostly devotional. They sing very beautifully, and here and there they say a few good things. There were no teachers here yet, so whoever came first was very popular, whether they were teaching the real and right things or not. If you do a little bit of exercise you'll feel better, so, of course these students say they felt many things with his practices. It's just the energy of their bodies beginning to move in a healthier way. He actually didn't talk about chakras much, and there are many sounds in the yogic systems that are missing from his teachings. Any kind of positive thinking can affect kundalini. Anyone who is teaching people to be positive in their life is teaching about kundalini in a way. To get the real benefits and create huge force in your kundalini, then you need to have the right techniques and the right guidance. Positive thinking cannot take you all the way by itself. Combined with learning how to dissolve karma and get rid of your toxins, it can take you closer to enlightenment, but he didn't teach those things. He didn't even know about the Tirthankaras, or real sadhana. He was more like a "Jehovah Witness" of Sikhism, and wanted to convert people. He was good in some ways. He inspired a lot of people to become vegetarian, and vegetarianism leads you to nonviolence, the first step of the spiritual path.

Sikhs don't really know what enlightenment is, the real thing. True yogis will never wear a turban. Unless they require it for a short time to be protected from weather or something. If Yogi Bhajan's students do the practices without wearing a turban, it will be much better for them. When you put a turban covering your head while practicing techniques to balance your chakras or awaken your kundalini, it can be very dangerous because you are blocking the energy and it might move to the wrong part of your body. Turbans have nothing to do with the yogic system. It is just part of the Sikh religion. A spiritual person will not wear it because it can block their energy if it's constantly on their head. Yogi Bhajan's students are unfortunately not aware that you shouldn't suffocate the chakras. At least take off the turban when you do practice. He has other beautiful teachings but people got stuck with what he mentioned about kundalini. It is better for them to do yoga or sing than perform his kundalini practices, because only yogis know the real system and Yogi Bhajan was not one of them. He was just an employee at an airport before he came to America.

You have to work really hard to raise your kundalini the right way, and if he was not even on the path how will he teach other people what to do? About kundalini awakening, people have a lot of misconceptions. They think if their energy is rising up to the seventh chakra, then they are enlightened. That is wrong. First thing, kundalini makes you just healthy, super healthy. But if you never get any further guidance from an enlightened person, you will never reach enlightenment, because you don't even have the right concept. Kundalini means you're making this instrument a little better to help you on the path of enlightenment, which is totally different.

When your kundalini is one day awakened 100%, you are in much better hands and can use your human body as the real instrument to go deep into meditation and be on the path. Enlightenment doesn't happen when your kundalini is 100% awakened, it is not sudden like that. There are many obstacles on the way that you have to overcome. Same way, if your kundalini is 50% awakened, it just means you are in good health, much better than most people. If you're lucky and get in touch with a real spiritual teacher, they can help you to be on the path. When healthy, you will not be negative, fearful or doubtful. You'll be able to receive the message more clearly. Many people do drugs and drink alcohol, and try to practice yoga on the side, but they don't have any guidance about the spiritual path. They continue to remain stuck.

Sometimes you can suddenly be shaken by your energy if you are hit or fall down in an accident, and the energy can be sped up. It goes through all the chakras, but it's sudden. When people go emotionally down, they sometimes get relaxed in their depression and their kundalini jumps in that relaxation. They might feel warmth or something, but they don't know what it is. If they feel it and there's no guidance to them from a master, then it doesn't even matter; they can't use it as an opportunity. So when people go to a yoga class and feel a little heat here and there, or some kind of sensation in the body, they think their kundalini is awakening. They are totally wrong. It is just the energy moving around and it feels good when the body is in motion and being active. That's all it is. People seem to have similar symptoms and experiences, but they are just mesmerized by something they have never felt before, and others might feel warmth somewhere and say the same things, that their kundalini must be awakening and amazing things are happening to them. It doesn't happen like that. It's not the real thing.

Karma can affect your kundalini in the sense that if you have light karmas left, the energy will automatically move a little bit faster and there are chances it will rise and take you to the path. Light karmas means there is a little less surrounding your soul and blocking your vision.

When the real kundalini awakening happens, it is very beautiful. That is the start of the path – when a person is really on the true path. You begin to look like a different person. Your eyes become more innocent and pure, and you'll become a very simple person. Not someone who wears a golden ring with a big sapphire in it like Yogi Bhajan. He met me once, and he said to me, "This sapphire, I can sell it for $150,000. That's in my ring." Those were his words to me. A yogi doesn't need luxury, and has no need to say those things. People are blind. What do yogis have to do with jewelry? His students are so blind they cannot even see what he was wearing.

When kundalini begins to rise in the real sense, the first symptom of awakening is the person will begin to leave their luxuries. They become like Mahavira or Buddha, very simple. They just need a little shelter and some food. Forget rings and jewelry, why do they need them? They will be simple, kind and forgiving, and become very healthy. Maybe they don't renounce right away, it might take them time to find the master or finish their responsibilities, but you will notice they suddenly become very simple. This is the beginning of the real kundalini awakening. It means they are moving towards the spiritual path.

The body becomes very healthy, and the mind will begin to cooperate with you when your kundalini begins rising. The body becomes fully at ease. If something is wrong in the body, it becomes diseased or in discomfort. It means the energy is not working the right way. Buddhists say, more or less, that all humans are mentally sick. Christians say we are all sinners. They are both in the same boat. Don't get trapped in it. They are teaching that if you're mentally sick, what will happen? If you're mentally sick, you cannot straighten out your sickness? If you're born as a sinner, what is the meaning of praying? An apple tree is born with sweetness; can you take away that sweetness? No; that is its nature. So can you take away the sins from someone who is born a sinner? They say come to Jesus and he will take away your sins. If you're born a sinner, then no one can take away your sins. Divinity can only produce divinity. You will never discover what God is if you believe you're a sinner.

Sometimes instead of going upward, the energy can go sideways in your body. This is very dangerous; it can make a person crazy, like an extreme vagabond or psychopath. These kind of people can be found all over Manhattan in New York City, or Haridwar in India. They get so stuck into something that their life loses its meaning. In India they call themselves sadhus but they are mostly crazy. Their energy went the wrong way completely. They smoke and do drugs, and I don't know why ignorant Hindus are worshipping them for. They don't get it; they even see them smoking marijuana or using hard drugs, and they still bow down in front of them. What can be more ignorant than this? People in India don't know what enlightenment really is. At least Yogi Bhajan taught not to drink, smoke or eat meat, but he was wrong to try and convert people.

When you give your energy to another person, it's called *shaktipat*. It works through your hands, but you don't need to be touching the other person. The real thing rarely happens. Sheep follow sheep. In those places, you can go to the T.V., like the Christian ministers that are healing people and they fall down to the floor. All those people are hired and they are paid very well. They're actors and they misguide all of these people right in front of them. They're not healing anybody. As soon as the person falls down, they catch them right away. It's all rehearsed ahead of time. Once in a while you can heal someone, like if they meet an enlightened person, their energy will begin to move, even if they don't talk to him or her. They just have to be near and see them.

A master doesn't need to touch. The person receiving doesn't even have to know the master did anything either. It can happen other ways, too. Maybe someone's first chakra is blocked and they come across an elephant and spend time near it, the chakra will begin to move a little bit. It won't move much, but it will affect it a little bit, because an elephant represents earth, the element of the first chakra, and also the fifth chakra's element is bone and the elephant has very big bones. It can happen when someone goes to the ocean, beach or river – anywhere there is water – because the element of the second chakra is water, so the energy will move a little bit. I will give more examples in relation to each chakra later. When you receive energy from a master, if you feel anything, it will be calm, peaceful, and relaxing. It will never make your body contort, twitch or make strange noises, like the "shaktipat" videos you can find on YouTube.

People who practice Reiki can just give their energy a little bit, if they even know how to produce it with the true technique. The way they do it comes from shaktipat. Reiki is shaktipat, but it's not done the right way. Whoever started this technique, went to India and saw shaktipat happen, not by sitting on a mountain, however their story goes. Buddha doesn't appear in front of anyone to give things. Because in Japan they are Buddhists, he said the Buddha gave him the technique in order to establish credibility of Reiki. Maybe if he said that Jesus showed him the technique, or Mohammed, the people wouldn't want anything to do with it. Reiki is shaktipat – just giving energy. They claim to know about the chakras and read auras. Sometimes there are people who become more like psychic fortune-tellers. People begin to ask them if they can see auras, and maybe they cannot, but because they see so many people they become a kind of expert in reading them. After a while they might see a few hundred people and they will see the same symptoms, and slowly by talking to them, they become experts. It's similar to a psychologist in that aspect. These people can collect a lot of bad karma by misguiding others. If they say that they see a bad color in someone's aura, but don't know what they're really looking at, the person can go down into a depression. If they inspire the people in some way, then they won't come back to ask for help and they are out of business then. They want people to come back so they can again collect more money.

I've met a lot of aura readers and reiki practitioners, and they haven't even changed their diets from eating meat and they call themselves spiritual. People using reiki or chakra healing cannot raise your kundalini. They can help you to take away a little discomfort but not much else. If you don't have money, suppose, how can you give it to someone else? If someone is sick, or very weak, how can they heal another person? If someone is weak and they try to heal someone or give them energy, all of that person's sickness can enter into the person trying to heal them. Many times the person doing reiki doesn't know how to protect themselves the right way. It is better not to put yourself in illusion. It's good to consider the doctor's opinion, because if a master sees that someone has cancer in an advanced stage, they know they cannot do anything to help it. What will a simple reiki practitioner do, if even an enlightened master cannot help? There are exceptions, but it is better to follow the opinion of trusted experts in some cases.

You need to make your body the healthiest in order to be on the path towards enlightenment, and kundalini, your energy, will make your body like that – very pure. We have the best instruments to realize our souls, but we don't have the knowledge about how they work. Our systems are very complex, and can be thrown out of balance by many things. If you want to be spiritual, you need to know the truth about your body first.

PRANA

Prana is a vital force. The sun gives us life, that is sure, but prana is totally different. We call it also pranic-force; many people know it as this. Pranic-force is all over, everywhere within our bodies, and by that force we are alive. The planet is alive because of the sun, but if we had an alternative then we actually don't need the sun. It is just a matter of technology. A person can be alive without the sun, but they cannot be alive without prana. Prana is life-force that is mixed with consciousness, because you have this body. All the pain, suffering, happiness, all sensations, these are all types of prana. There are ten main pranas, and they flow around every part of our bodies. Prana moves you, inspires you, does something for you, makes you happy, unhappy; this is all prana. Not only does it provide life and breath, it provides everything else, such as improving your chakras. These are the main ten pranas:

Sparsh indriya, touch, is the ability to feel sensations of touch. Is it hot or cold? Is it hard? Some sandpapers are rough, while some are more smooth. Without this prana you cannot feel things in this way.

Ras indriya, taste, is the ability to sense different tastes.

Ghran indriya, smell, is the ability to sense different smells.

Chakshu indriya, sight, is the ability to see all the things around you.

Shravan indriya, hearing, is the ability to hear.

Mano bala, mind, is the ability to think.

Vachan bala, speech, is the ability to speak.

Kaya bala, body, is the ability to move your body.

Shwasoshwas, respiration, is the ability to breathe.

Ayushya, longevity, is the ability to live.

Prana is coming from life, but life is not just one thing, like the sun giving us light. Prana comes from deep down in the subtle bodies. Our subtle bodies are alive. This physical body, is run by the subtle bodies. Subtle bodies are the real pranic-force. If the subtle bodies are not with this physical body, their house, then the physical body cannot be alive. Suppose the subtle body which is known as the fire body, the *Tejas* body, is not in the physical body, then it cannot create heat and it won't digest any food at all. If you go deep into meditation you can communicate with those bodies. They are the real bodies, not this physical body which we see and feel all the time. Behind those subtle bodies is a soul. If the soul is not connected with the subtle bodies, then the subtle bodies will disappear. But, as long you are living in this physical body it means the subtle bodies are there, too, because they carry your karmas that brought you to this body and this life.

Life doesn't come from the sun. The sun makes trees and plants grow, helps create wind, and we can harvest food and many other things because of the sun. We have life through the sun, but you can still grow things underground. There's no necessity of the sun. There are things like that underground. Sun is the main source for our planet, but it's not the ultimate source. You can be without it, but if you don't create the new source then of course you will need the sun still. If the sun is the source of prana, then everyone will have the same amount of prana, but it's not the case. Trees only have three *balpranas*: touch, age and breath. It breathes through its pores. The lowest category of life has only these three balpranas. When the senses increase, the pranas increase at the same time.

The soul has to evolve in order to gain the higher senses. When you get a body with five senses, like some animals, or a human, then you get *manbalprana*, a developed mind. Animals have a mind that is only slightly developed, but humans' minds are very developed, we can think about a lot of things and understand deeper things.

You have to understand that soul started from algae or amoeba. How much are they into the dark? They don't know anything about it. This is from beginning-less time. It is the combination of matter and soul. The glue came from the matter and the soul gets stuck in the karma. It's not real glue, because nothing can touch the soul. Soul is in the grip of karma, that's why it's in the dark. It hasn't yet gone through evolution; it hasn't improved. Only the soul who improves comes into a more developed life, such as a human-being or animal. Animals begin to think when they live with the human, otherwise they don't think. Like a tree, the tree has a main soul, but it doesn't think about anything, such as who is climbing or who's not climbing, or who's breaking the branches or who's not breaking the branches. They feel the sensation, but they don't know anything about it. They are in an unconscious state and do not know anything beyond what they feel.

The two-sensed living beings have a little awareness, because they eat at least and they can move; trees cannot even move. Only a few trees can go miles and miles, but they have to spread everywhere. The trees have seeds, and the seeds spread all over. They want to spread all over the world. It's not just humans that want to be everywhere, there are trees like that. They produce seeds and the wind will take them away. Wherever they go, they spread. So, those trees are a little improved comparatively to another type of tree, but they still don't have that consciousness that they can think yet, or feel pain. When a person is unconscious they don't feel pain.

So, the soul is in the grip of dirt, karma. Soul is pure, it doesn't have any dirt on it, it's in the grip of karma only. It's like the sun – shining. And the clouds are millions of miles from the sun. They don't touch the sun, but they still can block all the light. That is how matter works. Matter cannot touch the soul, because it's untouchable; it has no form or shape. Matter can go around it only, so it blocks the light. These *jivas*, living beings, are in the dark because of this. They haven't evolved yet or improved. Because they don't have manbalprana they aren't able to think about what's happening. They have to just go through natural evolution. It's hard to improve because there is no mind to decide what to do. It has to be natural only, which takes infinity to improve.

Suppose somebody has a strong piece of metal, a huge pillar, and you have just a tiny piece of sandpaper. Can you sand the whole pillar until it's gone? A little sandpaper and a huge pillar. Can you do it? That's how the natural way works. It takes so much time. That is evolution. Evolution happens slowly, very slowly. Charles Darwin was not right in that sense. He said that we come from monkeys and apes. That's what he called evolution. Evolution is not that. Evolution is, whoever is in the dark, an unconscious state, they slowly improve, but it takes infinity to improve. But once you get two senses, three senses, four senses, then you begin to improve a little bit quicker. Once you have five senses you can improve even more, because you can hear, see, taste, smell, feel and think. Animals can improve more, but humans? Humans can improve very quickly because of their developed mind. If they find the spiritual path they can improve so fast and burn their karma.

The only problem is how do you get on the spiritual path? Somebody has to inspire you, because if you're not inspired then you're just happy in your own cocoon. Nobody bothers you, you don't bother anybody, that's it. Some people are drunk all day, their parents left them millions of dollars. They have so much money but nothing to do, no inspiration. If they get inspired, then they can help a lot. Brad Pitt was inspired by Angelina Jolie. Though he did some charity work before he met her, he did not do as much as he does these days. She inspired him, and with President Bill Clinton they are all working together in New Orleans to help after the Hurricane Katrina disaster. People are still suffering there, they don't have homes. Brad Pitt always had the money, but he needed to be inspired to help a lot. So, now he begins to collect good karma and in his next life he'll begin to improve, even unknowingly. If he enjoys the charity and is whole-heartedly into it without expectation, then he will improve even more.

All living beings, jivas, have prana. No matter if they are a one-sensed living being like algae, a three-sensed living being such as an ant, or a more developed animal or a human with five senses. All living beings have prana because the pranic-force is in the subtle bodies that bring them into a body to begin with. When anything is alive they have prana. They have their own aura and subtle bodies. It's important not to step on algae because it has infinite living beings in it and infinite space. When it grows on top of water and becomes green, that kind of algae has a lot of life. They all have prana because they all have soul, and soul doesn't move in this world without subtle bodies.

Since the beginning, in the *Upanishadas*, where prana was first mentioned, they have only talked about the breath. All of the Hindu books mentioned it, but they mostly talked about the wind and air in the body.

That prana is just the airs in different parts of the body. The idea is not totally wrong, but they missed the whole concept. Breath is just one thing. We breathe through our nose or through our mouth, but the tree doesn't have either of these parts, but they still are breathing in a different way. They breathe through their pores. Breath is important, but it's just one prana.

Sometimes one or more pranas can be missing, like, if a person is born deaf, their vital force to hear is missing. Their shravan indriya prana is missing. It means there is very little or no prana to enable them to hear. Somebody has a mind, but they might have a disease that disables parts of their communication, maybe they think very slowly and cannot bring their words forth, it shows their mental prana is lacking. They may be intelligent in different ways, maybe they become artists, but their mind gives them trouble in thinking because the prana is not there. Sometimes people cannot smell, or they are blind or partially blind. This is vital force; through it we can see, we can hear, smell and so on. Through the *Purnam System*, which is a yogic system I created, you can increase the prana that you have. You will learn more about this system later. If you're born without the prana then you cannot do anything, that is sure, but if you have a little, you can increase what is already available.

There are five different pranas related to the breath only: *prana vayu, apana vayu, udana vayu, samana vayu* and *vyana vayu.* Prana vayu is the breath itself. Without it, you cannot be alive. When your breath stops somehow, then the physical body will also stop working; its purpose is to keep your body alive and working.

Apana vayu is the air that is below your diaphragm and stomach. It's below your navel near the second chakra. If something is wrong with this prana then you can get sick very easily. If a person cannot release this air from their body, it can create a poison inside. Food can go bad in your stomach because of the poison. In many people's cases, it doesn't work fully. It creates constipation, extreme violence and anger. It keeps a person in illusion. Naturally, this air flows downward, but if for some reason it begins to flow upward, a person can die. You never want this prana to flow upward in the body. Apana also means downward. This apana vayu keeps you healthy.

Three leshyas, intentions, as taught by the 23rd Tirthankara, Parshvanath, are related to the apana vayu: Krishan, Neel and Kapota. These are mostly the lower leshyas, the lower intentions. When somebody is in the Krishan leshya, they feel violent and heavy. When in the Neel leshya, they're a little less heavy, but emotionally down, never feeling happy. Kapota is the same also but a little lighter. These people are not very positive, and their sexual energy is very active so they think negatively. It is all related to the prana, because it affects the whole body, and if it's heavy the senses cannot work properly and the emotions and thoughts are affected a lot.

Udana vayu is connected from the heart up to the head, and it flows upward in the body, not downward. It can clear all of your senses. If udana vayu is flowing downward, it can also be possible for the person to have a lot of sicknesses and die.

Samana vayu is a balance between udana and apana vayu. It's in the center part of the body and relates to the third chakra. If there is a problem here, a person will not be stable or balanced. It can create that situation where you suddenly go into *turiyam*, consciousness, but the pranas have to be working properly together. This vayu helps to digest the food in your system. Udana vayu flows upward, apana vayu flows downward and samana vayu is balanced in the center. It can take you into the *Sushumna* channel, the main nadi or nerve, where it's possible to enter into meditation.

Vyana vayu is all over the body, everywhere. Vyana means "spread all over." Its purpose is to keep you very healthy. If the vyana vayu doesn't move well in your hand, then it will create a lot of pain in your hand, or somewhere else that isn't working well. If all of these are balanced the right way and have good coordination together, you can enter into meditation then.

Shwasoshwas prana is the breath. You breathe in and you exhale. This is your life, and it's the fire throughout your entire body to burn all the toxins and karma. If you want to awaken your kundalini and open all of your chakras then you need to raise your intention out from the lower three leshyas into the Padma leshya and up to Shukal leshya. If you have a low pranic-force in your system then you will stay in the lower leshyas. Your chakras will be stuck and have no current to take you higher. People who have the lowest prana are very violent, they can attack people or have outbursts of rage, become rapists or sexually abuse children. You don't want to be this low, so work on your body, work on your thoughts; make them pure. Eat the best foods for your body while doing minimal harm and your prana will be very healthy and light. Automatically your chakras and kundalini will be in better hands before you begin your sadhana.

Our bodies have complex systems, I mentioned, so you have to take care of them to keep everything clear. When your nadis are clear, prana can flow equally, and when it flows equally you are healthy. Chinese people call prana, "chi," but it is referring to the same energy. Tai Chi helps in the same way yoga does, but it's an imitation of yoga and a very slow process. It doesn't happen quickly. The Purnam System is very fast to increase chi, or prana, in the body. When I teach the Purnam Yoga retreats at Siddhayatan, the students always feel an immediate change and shift in energy. They feel lighter. When your nadis are clear the energy can move efficiently through the body, your chakras will be more balanced and you'll have chances to go into meditation, into deep consciousness.

In that space you will find many beautiful things; you will begin to see the soul. Prana originates from the subtle bodies, and they are full of information, including all of your karma. They are full of karma. Full of fire. Full of light. When they begin to empty, that is when you can see glimpses of your soul. But, if they remain full of information then the soul will never wake up. It will be dragged from this life to another life, another place, and so on, never ending. The subtle bodies take your soul here and there because of all the information they carry. All your karmic information is recorded in them, and until they are dissolved and no information remains in the subtle bodies then you'll continue in the cycle of birth and death, suffering, changing, everything constantly going up and down, up and down. Wherever subtle bodies go, soul has to follow because it's very weak. They drag the soul around until you work on yourself and the soul begins to slowly realize its power. When the soul gets power, then the subtle bodies have no power. Soul is separate from prana. If you're born with ten pranas, but one or two prana die somehow, then you can still be alive. Unless you lose your breath, swashoswash, then that is a different story. You cannot live without breath. Sometimes you can't even eat, you are on life support. It seems like even if you're lacking some of the pranas then you are still all right. The soul can still stay there in the body.

A human is supposed to be born with the ten main prana, the balpranas, but, sometimes a person is born lacking half of them. They are still a human. If you have an accident and go blind, it means you lost that prana. You no longer have chakshu indriya. Diseases, too. If you have aayu balprana, age, then you will go on a life-support system and continue living no matter how many other pranas you lose. You'll live until the aayu balprana prana runs out. All of your prana has to die before your physical body can die. If a person is blind or deaf, sometimes both, they can still be a very good singer. Sometimes a person who loses prana can gain more strength through the remaining prana. One is missing, but power comes to the other prana and they are very talented. It happens in some cases. Stevie Wonder plays incredibly, but he is blind, so, his other pranas became stronger.

Subtle bodies exist because the soul is weak. When the body dies and a person is liberated, then the subtle bodies are empty and can't drag you anywhere. Maybe your computer chip is full of information, but you delete it accidentally. It doesn't mean it's gone, you can find it and recover it somehow. You might have to spend a lot of money to send it to a specialist who can get it back, but it is still there. Once the subtle bodies are empty, it is not like the computer chip; they are fully empty. That is when soul is liberated. Nobody can reach liberation when they commit suicide or die, otherwise everyone would be liberated. Liberated souls don't have prana, they are just soul. Soul has no source to get light. Soul is light. It's infinite; it never ends. It has no source of light, but it is light. Suppose you have a battery and it charges by itself, no source needed – no solar power, no electricity or plugs. It's not a complete example, but the soul is like that, with no source. The light doesn't come from somewhere. A candle has a source, and a light bulb has a source. When you light the candle you see where the light is coming from. When you turn on a light-switch, you know the light is coming from the electricity, it's why you have to turn the switch. Soul is not like that.

When a person's pranic force is low, it means the air in the body, the five vayus, is not flowing equally in the different parts of the body. Whatever is eaten will get stuck in the intestines and they can get sick all the time and have a weak body. If one prana is off balance, others are off balance, too. Samana vayu needs to balance them. That's why we say the third chakra, *Manipura*, is very important. You'll learn more about the Manipura in Part III; for now, it's the axle of the body, the center. It's connected with the solar system. Because of the sun we don't have to seek other kinds of energy. Dizziness, heaviness, pain, a lot of diseases can happen when we have low pranic-force. If a person has fear all the time, they should eat light food and change what foods they're eating. It will help a lot. When a person has low prana it will take a year to two years to pick up and create a lot of energy, but if they are determined and they really want it, then they can do it.

NADIS

In this body, we have nerves running everywhere. They take messages to the brain where we can use our mind to pick apart the information. We have three main nerves; they are known as nadis in the yogic system. *Nadi* means "nerve." Main nerves function well if they are clear; the blood will flow equally. They carry the vital things that our body needs. These are physical and have structure – our veins, arteries, nerves, and so on – these are all nadis.

Remember, in order to get the full benefits of spirituality and the entire chakra system you need to know about your body, the way it works, and how to purify it. When the nadis are blocked by toxins, our bodies will have trouble functioning how they're supposed to. Our brain won't get the right messages from our central nervous system with these toxins in the way, and in turn our physical and mental health are affected greatly. Maybe these toxins are creating some kind of problem with the circulation of blood in your body because of fat build-up from unhealthy foods or some other cause. It will give you a lot of pain and discomfort, and can be very bad for your organs and heart, among other things. How will your thoughts be if you are constantly in discomfort from these ailments? It is very difficult to keep yourself in positive thoughts, spiritual thoughts, when your body is not healthy. A healthy body is required on the spiritual path. All of these things relate to the chakras, because it affects the energy in your body; it affects your thoughts, and your emotions will always be down if your body is giving you discomfort every day.

Out of all of these nadis, there are three that we have to pay special attention to: *Ida nadi*, *Pingala nadi* and *Sushumna nadi*. Ida nadi keeps our body's temperature regulated at a cool level. It's also known as the *Chandra nadi*; the moon channel. If there is no breath flowing in this nadi, due to a blockage, then the temperature can increase up to 500 degrees. You will burn alive inside.

The Pingala nadi keeps you warm and balances the heat in your body so you don't freeze. You can freeze to death if there is no breath flowing in this nadi. *Surya nadi*, sun channel, is another name for the Pingala nadi.

The third nadi, Sushumna, is the most important. It keeps you balanced; your body doesn't burn, and it doesn't freeze.

Swashoswash prana, breath, flows through the nadis. The breath is just one prana, remember. Without the main prana you are not conscious. When there is prana you feel it – pain, happiness, sadness, all of these things. Consciousness doesn't flow in the nadis. If the pranas are equal, if they're balanced and the nadis are all the way clear, then you can jump into the consciousness through the Sushumna nadi. You can, but it's not the purpose. The main purpose of the nadis is for prana to flow in the body.

First, our brain has so many blood vessels and they need to be provided with the cleanest blood. Whatever we're eating and drinking, if it's not healthy, light food, what our bodies need, then the blood will not be pure and it begins to block the nadis by creating little clogs and build-ups here and there. It prevents the healthy blood from getting where it needs to go throughout the brain, so our mental processes are affected in a big way. Maybe right now we think we are healthy, we think that we eat the best food, but the impurities in our blood don't come only from our current life. They are brought with us from life to life, collecting more and more impurities by our karma. Being healthy doesn't mean to simply eat good foods; you have to understand what your own body requires, and how it is affected. You have to clean your blood and your whole system with yogic techniques. Pranayama is just one way to do this. When the nadis are clogged here and there, we think more on the negative side, on the heavy side. It doesn't mean you are negative all the time, every day. Maybe you have a lot of success in your life but you are too hard on yourself or others, maybe you don't see all the sides of something. So, if you know how to unblock them and keep them clean all the time, you can become completely healthy, and health leads to enlightenment. A sick person cannot become enlightened.

How do they become blocked? If you're not aware about eating and drinking, like, you eat or drink bad things, use alcohol, contaminated water, heavy foods all the time, lots of oily or greasy food, fried foods, then your nadis become blocked right away with many toxins. No matter what you do, you cannot achieve your goals. Whatever you want in your life, you'll have many obstacles just in your mind and body alone, forget about the outside things. By using drugs, alcohol and other things that can really harm your body, they not only block the nadis, but they can damage them beyond repair. You will have a hard time to breathe the right way, to breathe clearly. Once the nadis are damaged like this they cannot be repaired by any kind of practices. When we are working on our bodies we want to remain in good health and have no risks. You never want to touch these things like alcohol, or cigarettes, marijuana, LSD – never do it. By cleaning the nadis, we become balanced and the temperature in our body is equal. Food is digested right away and there will be no big problems. This is the way to meditation, with good health.

The center nadi, Sushumna, is inside the backbone. It's the main channel in the body. Sushumna helps you remain balanced. If you understand why, it can help you a lot on your path. When only the Ida nadi is open you are in your emotions too much. The Ida nadi is the main nerve running on the left side of your body. Ida means moon. This is the channel that helps to cool you down. When the Ida is open, and the Pingala is blocked too much, you may cry often or feel very upset. It means something is blocking the Pingala nadi, so your breath is flowing only in the Ida nadi. Your breath stays in the Ida nadi when you inhale and exhale, and it builds up and creates a coolness. The air stays in that side of your body and creates imbalance. You become very emotional.

Just the opposite, when the Ida is mostly closed and the Pingala nadi is open, you may be more jealous, angry, too proud, greedy, these kinds of things. It creates more heat in you when the Pingala is more open than the Ida. Pingala runs on the right side of your body, and it's known as the sun channel. Meditation will happen only when we are not in those emotions, when we are in the third channel, Sushumna. It means we are balanced already, and it helps to go into meditation. You're steady, focused, concentrated. You can work without getting tired. If the nadis are not balanced, everything will happen. Emotions will attack us more and bring us down when we're in the Ida or Pingala nadi. Sushumna is the passage and energy flows through it. Once the nadis are clear the energy can flow very easily and you'll be able to balance your chakras much quicker.

In the *Upanishadas*, very old texts from India, they say there is one artery that goes from the heart to the crown of the head, and at the time of death it's the way you become immortal. They also believe that there are five divine holes located in the heart, called *shushis*, through which the divine can be perceived. These shushis are somehow connected to the seventh chakra. What they are referring to is not really an artery, it seems more like the Sushumna, where the prana flows in a balanced way. When you are balanced you can see clearly. They say in Hinduism that soul lives only in the heart, but I disagree. Soul lives everywhere in the body, not just the heart. They say it may be because the heart is the main organ in the body to pump blood. It's an important part of the body, but it doesn't mean soul lives there. You can make an artificial heart now, anyway. If you take out the person's heart and replace it with an artificial one, soul is still there. It's not in the heart. You have to put efforts and work really hard in purifying your nadis.

It's not just simple stuff, like reading about it and then it happens, no. You have to do a lot of work. Nowadays some people try to relate a lot of astrology to the nadis, like reading your nadi leaves. Those nadis have nothing to do with the real system. All our breath flows through your nervous system, and this is different. Those people think they can read you, but it's the same thing if you go to the psychologist. They are experts on how to talk to you. They hear the same problems again and again, the same questions. They might try to tell you many things are happening, they see symptoms repeated from other people and learn what to say. None of it is real. Nadis are in our body and totally different from these people claiming to read nadis. We need to keep them clear and unblocked, so our kundalini can flow and our chakras can be awakened.

AURAS

Many people are curious about the aura. Everyone has this aura, no matter if it's a human, an animal, a plant, bacteria, or something else. All living beings have an aura. If you know how to see them you can see what kind of person is in front of you by looking at distribution of the light. Six months before a person dies, their aura begins to shrink. It becomes smaller and smaller; it's a sign that they won't survive more than six months. On the planets where angels are born, they know when their death is coming close because they have that vision to see the aura. It is up to us if we want to know it. You can see them if you are sensitive.

You have to know that the aura is separate from the subtle bodies. They are not the same thing, don't be confused about it. The subtle bodies are inside the physical body, they have their own colors but they are a different thing. When the subtle bodies leave the physical body, when they travel, the aura stays with the physical body.

Depending on the state of each chakra, how healthy the energy is, they create different colors in the aura and the intensity of the light – how bright the colors appear. If the colors are more dim and not shining, it means there's a problem in the chakras. Kundalini is not flowing the right way.

The aura reveals what kind of person you are. Suppose someone has a lot of white light in their aura, they will be very serene, clear-minded, live in a healthy way and have positive thoughts. If black is more visible, then they may be a more negative person, or maybe they want to be positive but they struggle with themselves in their mind a lot and have jealousy and anger. When red is the strongest color it indicates the person has a lot of energy, a lot of mental activities, but they don't know how to use the energy to their benefit. If the person is really on the path you can suggest how to use their energy the right way, but I don't recommend saying those things. Every color has a different meaning and the brightness, too.

To see the aura, you have to go deep into meditation. First, you have to learn what meditation means; you need a lot of concentration and focus. The best thing to do is practice *tratka*, a technique from many thousands of years ago. It will help your concentration tremendously. It is very simple and anybody can practice this technique. If you have glaucoma, or other troubles with your eyes I don't recommend practicing it. Do not practice in a room or open space with wind or other moving air; it can damage your eyes.

Find a piece of white paper, and in the center make a black circle and fill it in with black ink. The circle needs to be about one inch in diameter, the size of a quarter-dollar coin in the United States. What you do is place this sheet of paper on the wall in front of you, level with your eyes, and sit 12-18 inches away from it. Keep your eyes open and stare at the center of this black circle. The black circle on the white paper is important, because the contrast does something to your eyes. Maybe in the beginning you can only stare for five or ten seconds before the pain is too much and you have to close your eyes. Do it again and again, increasing your time with each practice. Try to make it to one minute, then two minutes. Whatever stress you feel in your eyes, try not to blink. They will twitch and move and sting as they become dry. Eventually you'll be able to hold them open long enough that tears begin coming down from your eyes. After you have a lot of practice you can try to stare for 10 minutes, 15 minutes, or even 30 minutes, 40 minutes and up to an hour.

This practice will give you tremendous strength. All the power comes into your eyes when you do this technique. If you can sit or stand, without blinking at all and keeping your body still while you stare, all the consciousness in your body flows into your eyes and you gain a lot of power. Your thoughts will stop attacking you when the mind realizes you won't pay attention to them. Your body will be relaxed and you'll feel a wave of calm in your body. This is the power you need to concentrate in meditation.

After you practice tratka, you have to work on visualization. Strong visualization takes a lot of practice; it is different from tratka. Tratka is just for concentration. To practice visualization, go into a very dark room at night. Place a candle eight feet in front of where you will stand or sit. Stare at the candle's flame for 30 seconds and then close your eyes. You'll see the flame remaining there with your eyes shut. Maybe just for one or two seconds before it disappears. Stare at the flame again and try to reach 45 seconds. This time it might stay in your vision for a few more seconds. Practice this every day, trying to stare at the flame for five minutes, and maybe after 21 days if your visualization is gaining strength you can walk into the same room and when you close your eyes the candle will be there even without lighting it. If you had Lasik surgery then it is not a good idea for you to stare at the flame, but tratka is okay.

That is visualization. It can be expanded to anything. People don't know how to heal someone from far away. When you have a strong visualization you can think about the person and bring them into your vision. They might be thousands of miles away from you, but you can see them clearly. Concentrate on the area where they have pain or some kind of problem, on the area of visualization. It is actualization. Actualization is when your visualization becomes stronger and stronger. It's not that you bring the person to you. Your subtle body travels to them and it can heal the person sometimes. When you have that kind of visualization, that's when you begin to see the real aura. Otherwise you cannot be sensitive. It is light. After that it simply happens; you begin to see the light around the person or animals or other living beings. Then you need further knowledge about what the colors mean, and how the light is moving. First, be strong in concentration and then move to visualization.

If you're familiar with a person and you can see their aura is beginning to shrink, like it is not as big as before, then you can know they will die soon. Otherwise, if you don't know the person or have a lot of experience looking at the aura you won't be able to understand what it's doing. You can warn the person to be healthy, more spiritual; you don't tell them exactly they are going to die, because they will die even quicker. You never say negative things like that. Sometimes, I know a person is going to die the next day, I never tell them, because they will get so shocked that they'll die in one hour. Sometimes it is better to not tell truth.

Every kind of angel is into luxury, because where there is so much pleasure on those planets they don't know what spirituality means. Their lives are luxury, nothing else. They cannot see spirituality. If there is no up and down in life, you don't think about spirituality or try to find meaning in life. But they have the vision to see auras at far distances and many things, so they see their aura shrinking and know what it means. They will get sad because they know they will lose their luxuries and pleasures, and soon have to go to the next birth and have a dirty stomach and organs and these things. They have avadhi jnana and can see where they will go. They begin to focus on the family where they'll be born. They begin to put positive energy into that family to help them have more positive thoughts if they're not living in a good way, to clean themselves and take responsibility for things. When the aura begins to shrink, the subtle bodies don't exit. Subtle bodies are there, but they leave in the end, just before the death. All the particles of the soul and subtle bodies begin to form a line to the womb where they will go into the body. A direct line from wherever their planet is, to the planet where they will be born, and all the particles begin to go there. In the last moment when they lose breath, that is when the last particles go – the moment of conception.

Our auras will protect us if the white light is strong. White light is protective light. It will give you vision, like not to go here, or not to do that thing. If you're driving, it will make you think not to drive too fast, or not to turn at that moment. You will get some kind of indication like that, but it doesn't mean you will even notice it or listen to it if you do, it's up to you. But that happens only when we have a lot of white light in our auras.

The best way to create this protection in the beginning is to become very strong in visualization. Every morning, you close your eyes and visualize bright white light surrounding your entire body, entering you and covering you. All day it will help you. You have to be an expert in visualization first, you have to see the light all around you. So, if you're with negative people or anything like that, your chakras won't be affected by them, or your moods won't go up and down from hearing negative things or reading them, seeing them, and so on.

If you want to try and feel the aura you can try a simple way. If you're in a group of people, stand in a circle all holding eachother's hands. Everyone has to close their eyes and let go of their thoughts, be very relaxed. You'll begin to feel some kind of energy. It flows from one person to another. If there is only you and one other person, bring your hand to the other person's hand. Sometimes you can feel there is a kind of current between the hands, even without touching. If you're sensitive enough you can see a haziness around the fingers, like a glow or a cloud. That is part of your aura. Anyone can try these techniques, it doesn't matter if they are spiritual or not, because energy can be felt by anyone. The aura is energy, so they will feel its warmth and they might get a little idea that spirituality is something to think about.

The first layer of the aura is called *pratham abhavrita*, it means the first circle, or first layer of the body. It's a light body, like space, and it's empty. You can also call it the etheric body. There's nothing in it. Only *darmastikaya* particles, so it can move. There are no *adarmastikaya* particles. If you go into space, you will keep going and going because there are no adarmastikaya particles; they help you to stop. On Earth, we have both kinds of particles, so if you're walking you can stop if you choose. This first layer of the aura cannot stop its movement, so if you don't have control, then what is going to happen is the etheric body will go here and there, and you don't have the force to bring it back. Even though it's good that it has movement around you, if your aura is not strong the first layer might be released and there is no protection.

This layer is a circle, a quarter inch up to two inches away from the body. If you put your hands near your skin you'll feel some kind of energy or sensation there. It is light around your body. Its color is a light bluish-grey, and it has a kind of pulse, 15-20 cycles in each pulse. If a person comes to you and you look at their shoulders, you'll see a dark color. If you touch it or put your hand there, you'll feel the pulsation. You can see if the person is going forward or backward based on the color. This light bluish-grey is the color of the Neel and Kapota leshya. So, by seeing how bright the colors are you can check how their intentions are. Is it bright and shining, or dim and fading? If it's brighter then it means the person is improving themselves and going upward. If it's faded, it means the person is thinking negatively and going downward.

All light has structure. All light has particles. It's not just one light, it's all the particles floating around. Those light particles ride on other particles and things become visible. When there are particles, it means something has structure. This is why the aura can increase and decrease. This first layer, pratham abhavrita, is like a shining web of light, like beams of light. You can see the constant motion in this layer, constantly moving around in a clockwise circle. It is fully structured, like the physical body. Because it is so close to the physical body, you can see tissues, bones and organs through it. When you see this bluish-grey color is very strong around a person it means they are very sensitive and have a sensitive body, too. If they touch someone they feel a little shock. There are many people like this. You can see also, sometimes, from the shoulders and down the arms, it can be plain white or plain black, then it goes down the arms and becomes a bluish-grey. I see this sometimes. By looking at all the layers of the aura together, you can determine how healthy someone's body is. If this first layer is dim, then it means that person is about to get sick or develop a disease.

Dvitiya abhavrita is the second layer of the aura, sometimes called the emotional body. It carries all the feelings of a person. This layer extends from the body about 1-3 inches, and has a dark, muddy color. It has all the colors of the rainbow, but it is usually muddled, because when there are emotional problems and struggles, the person has dark spots here and there among the colors. They appear like broken circles, because this layer doesn't have definite structure, and is more fluid-like. It means the aura wants to float more, they're in motion more and want to be active. They have a sort of current that moves around freely like liquid. This is a person's kapot leshya. It means the person is coming out of the dark, slowly coming out of their ignorance, and making their intention higher towards spirituality.

Tritiya abhavrita is the name of the third layer, and it controls your thoughts and mental processes. This is the mental body, and usually visible near the head and shoulders first. It then radiates from there, all over the body. Its color is mostly yellow, full of ideas and thoughts, and has structure in it. When you can see a lot of yellow near the head and shoulders it means the person is really strong in thinking, analyzing, and being in their head. You'll usually see it beginning at 3-8 inches away from the body depending on it's strength. You can touch this layer if you're sensitive enough to see it. This is called Padma lesha. Having yellow light around your head and shoulders makes your intentions more pure, and you become wise.

The fourth layer of the aura is called *chaturtha abhavrita*, and it's known as the astral body, because it reflects how strong a person's subtle bodies are to communicate with other planets and enlightened people. This layer just reflects the strength of the astral body. It is fluid-like and can be seen 6-12 inches from the body. It floats around the body and has a beautiful rose color, usually. You see many people flowing in this color, because it extends to 12 inches away from them, it can strike on another person if they're close enough and they might get confused that the other has feelings of love for them. They begin thinking like that. It's not an actual indication of how the person feels, it is more like a little touch of energy and they can get into fantasizing love, not like real love. People begin to think that the other person wants them and it creates a lot of dilemma. This is called Tejo leshya. Its red color not only makes you active in love and compassion, but can also help you improve your intention to realize what God is and who you are. It brings you that much deeper inside yourself.

Next, the etheric template body is the fifth layer. It is not the real name, but people call it that. It is called *paṁcham abhavrita*. Usually it will begin around the fifth chakra, at the throat, and can be felt 18-24 inches from the body. It has a structure, but the problem is the color is absent. It is hard to describe if you cannot see it, but it seems like a negative of a photograph. It seems more like empty space, like when you see heat coming off of the horizon and it moves like that. There isn't really a color in this layer. When this layer is stronger, the person is going more upward now. It has a narrow, oval-like shape around the body. When it's very strong, the way a person speaks, it seems like they have unconditional love.

The sixth layer of our aura is called *shashtham abhavrita*, and it's very important. It's the celestial layer and can be seen two feet away from the body, almost to three feet away. This is the emotional level of the spiritual plane, but it's different from the second layer of the aura. It has no structure and consists of light, like shimmering beams. It's a kind of pastel, creamy color and has strong beams of light. When you see a candle and it has a glow around it, we call it *vrita*, in Sanskrit. The candle has its own glow, it gives you an idea of the aura. That's why we call the aura vrita. This layer has a big role because it takes you to the spiritual plane, from the emotional level of the spiritual plane, the higher emotions. You can jump from emotional to spiritual, like better emotions, but more on the spiritual side. When your heart chakra is fully open, no blockages at all, you can see this body more.

Saptam abhavrita is the causal body, the seventh layer of the aura. Its shape is egg-like around the body, a little bit wider than the fifth layer. I see that it's like gold and silver light, but not beams or solid colors; it's like thousands and thousands of shining gold threads all moving around each other within this layer. Tiny threads. Beyond this level is just the cosmic plane, and after that there is no other thing. It's everything around us, not what's part of our body. Our body is the seven layers, then after that it is very hard to explain the things in the cosmic plane. The saptam abhavrita can be seen four feet away from the body, and has structure. Some people think that this causal layer records all the memories and experiences the soul has gone through. It does, but in a different way. It's not like memories. It can expand up to 4 feet around the body, so it can fit a lot of things, and the strength of this layer, the brightness, it shows the kind of person it is because of the experiences their soul has had, but not like memories or pictures. It shows a general idea of what they have gone through.

Our aura changes colors constantly. Suppose you wake up angry, then one hour later your anger passes and you feel peaceful. It is going to change colors because the anger is momentary; all the emotions are momentary. As soon as one emotion dissolves or lessens, then the aura will appear different. It changes according to thoughts and emotions. All day long it changes constantly.

We want our auras to be very bright, very colorful, shining. That is the goal. All the subtle bodies are very healthy, and the brighter your aura is and more colorful, that's the best because it shows that everything is very healthy: spiritually, mentally and physically. An enlightened master's aura is mostly white, but all the colors are also there, too. They just may not be as strong.

An enlightened master's aura can extend for thousands of miles. People can be protected by it, even if they don't know that he or she is there. Sometimes the master cannot protect because something happens too quickly while they are busy doing something else. They might not make it in time. If there is a little time though, even a few seconds, they can protect the person. If there is a car accident, maybe the car will be smashed but the person doesn't die. Don't think God doesn't help you; God helps you all the time, but unknowingly. They don't know why they escaped without harm, just at the last moment. The master's aura can push you suddenly and you will get out of the way, or be in a better position. If you're closer to where a master is, then the protection is even stronger. If I meet you personally, because of the connection, I can protect you easily.

Our energy is mostly released through our feet, but it can enter anywhere in the body. Of course the head will feel it first because the mind and brain are there, so you'll notice the difference. We don't point our feet at someone we respect. The big toe is the biggest energy releaser, and you can lose all your energy when you point your feet at someone. It's different if you're moving, like walking outside. It doesn't drain much. Actually, when you stand on a big rock, or soil, earth, grass, things like this, you can gain energy, but when you stand on metals it drains faster than anything else. If you have socks on or shoes, then it mostly blocks receiving and draining both, but still it will drain if you stand on metals. When you are facing a master, like if you're sitting and listening to them talk and you have your legs pointed out towards them, their energy cannot be drained. A master is always protected, so they don't need to do anything. If someone is pointing their feet at a master it will actually drain their own energy faster than if they point their feet at someone on their own level. It is better not to point your feet at someone you respect, especially a master. The third-eye and hands suck in energy the most, so in India that's why it's a tradition to touch a master's feet with your forehead or hands, to get some energy for the day. You can even get a little shock, but only a little. It keeps you in positive thoughts and good feelings for the day. It's not permanent, and the next day you won't notice anything. In the crowds, a real master won't allow it. It will take all day, hours and hours if there is a big crowd of people. The real master won't want to waste so much time with that, and they would rather bless the people from a distance. If you're in a big crowd of people with a master it's better to just get the blessing from far away, even if others are touching their feet.

There is no need to touch even. Especially when you're trying to heal someone. I always suggest that people touch as less as possible when trying to heal someone. You don't need to put your hands right on them, it doesn't make the energy stronger. You can heal someone the same way even from five feet away. It's better because especially if the person is sick, or a negative person, then you protect yourself by not directly touching their body. And I recommend only to do it for 30 seconds, it's enough. There's no need to put your hand for 10 minutes.

Amritanandamayi in India is supposed to know this. She is widely known as "Amma, the hugging saint." She hugs everyone in the crowd. Sometimes four or six hours go by; she will go through the whole crowd to hug everyone. One time, a big group of people came to me after meeting her, and they said they waited all day to hug her, and they didn't feel anything when it finally happened. Of course not. She won't do anything. But by waiting four hours there, it's a kind of discipline and you are in positive thoughts with all the excitement and other people there, and that can heal you, not her hugs. You get the healing by doing it yourself, she cannot do anything. Hugging everyone is just more like to show it. She is not supposed to spend so much time in the crowd like that, she lacks the right knowing.

PURNAM YOGA

We can affect our chakras in many ways, both intentionally and unintentionally, knowingly and unknowingly. All of our surroundings can potentially create changes in our system, in turn yielding chaos such as diseases, mental and emotional unrest, uncertainty, confusion, or on the other hand, benefits such as harmony and balance within our inner-workings – necessities to deepen our spiritual understanding and expand our consciousness. In any moment you can see something with your eyes, or hear something in passing, and be affected in countless ways. It starts right where you are, with the society we live in. All these toxins in the body that we put over a long period of time, from our tensions and stress, the way we live and things we eat and drink, they keep us from being natural, from being free. If we want our chakras to be fully open, balanced, and our kundalini to rise up like the cobras in the Himalayas, then we need to purge these toxins out of our systems.

Purnam Yoga is a system that was realized sitting on top of the Himalayas, when I was doing intensive sadhana. It just happened naturally, and revealed itself in deep meditation. It was almost 150 years ago. Many postures and movements came to me while I was in that meditation. A figure came in front of me, in my vision, to do this posture and that posture, breathing in certain ways. It happened all by itself.

Purnam Yoga is more for health, because it can finish sickness in the body fully. Purnam means "perfect." The human body is the best instrument to grow spiritually, the only instrument. There are many things blocking it from being the healthiest body, but the Purnam System can get rid of all of these blockages and you can then blossom through your instrument. If you're not healthy, then there is no connection between your body and spirituality. A sick body cannot follow spirituality at all. In this aspect, Purnam is for health and spirituality, because it will create that kind of energy in your body that will help you advance on your spiritual path.

Your chakras open very quickly when you practice the Purnam System, because it's a divine system that cleans all of our channels. When the channels are clean, the energy begins to move upwards freely. If you have a fire and it's burning just a little bit, that is like the fire inside of you when you practice chakra techniques. But what happens when you take fuel and put it all over that little fire? It becomes a big, raging fire, and burns very quickly and strongly. When you practice the Purnam System at the same time as working on your chakras, you are throwing fuel onto your fire. It helps your chakras balance much faster.

Your aura will become much brighter, too. The aura has all of the colors, so automatically when the auras colors are very heavy and dim, there is something wrong in the body. After Purnam Yoga and breathing, throwing out all of the toxins, all the colors in the body become balanced and much brighter. Colors are already there, but they become shining and beautiful.

What happens when you practice the Purnam System is that you become dizzy or nauseated. It's the toxins that have never moved before, now they begin to move and they create some kind of illusion in front of you. You get dizzy. The brain and senses begin to live with those toxins all around them, and even though they are very harmful, you don't notice them because you have gotten used to them for so long.

Once, a king wanted a saint to live with him in his palace.

The monk said, "I cannot live in your palace. I smell gold there."

"I never smelled any gold," the king said, but the monk insisted he could not live there.

"How do you know it smells?" he asked the monk.

The monk took the king to an area near the coast where all the residents were fisherman. It was a fishing community, and they survived off of their catches from the sea. They were cutting fish everywhere, and as soon as the king entered with the monk, he covered his nose and complained so much to the monk.

"Where is it you're taking me? The smell is unbearable."

The monk told him to have a little patience, because he was also there smelling the same things. He talked to a couple of people, and the king mentioned there was such a big smell. They asked the king what he was talking about.

"I lived here for 40 years, and I never smelled anything that you talk about."

The king called over a couple of ladies and asked them the same thing. They also never smelled it in their whole life. It doesn't exist for them because their brain and body are adjusted to the smell. The king suddenly realized. He lives in the palace, so he doesn't smell the gold. He understood. When you live with something, it disappears from you. The brain becomes confused when these toxins finally move, even if it's just one or two layers of toxins. We live with the toxins but we don't notice them until they move around; the brain gets a little confused and we feel very dizzy as they begin moving.

Purnam Yoga moves all these layers of toxins. One-by-one. It shakes them out of their place and you expel them from your system with intense breathing during the postures and movements. Your nervous system becomes very active and will begin to send the right messages to your brain. If your nervous system is dull and slow, full of toxins, then it will always give you the wrong message. The first thing in the body to send the message is the nervous system, and they go first to the senses, and further. As soon as you do Purnam Yoga, the nervous system is opened and clear, more active, stronger, and you begin to receive the right message – the truth. Maybe you touch something hot and it feels cold; this can happen if your nervous system is not healthy. It's giving you the wrong message. When you clear your nervous system completely, it will be impossible for anybody to perform hypnotism on you, because you can see through it, you know what's really happening.

Your brain will become very sharp. There are certain practices in the Purnam System that increase your ability to learn because they clear your head out fully. I always say that the human is like an upside down tree. The tree has its roots in the ground, but the humans' roots are in the head. Our roots are not nourished and remain unclear, and toxic. This is why the brain doesn't work very well. Common people's brains work very little, because they're full of toxins; negative thoughts, jealousy, violence, they're all in the head, not in the heart. The more you practice the Purnam System, these things are thrown out of you forever. The brain will function very well and the IQ will increase on it's own.

Your skin will become like a baby's skin after some time of practice. All the toxins are out – thrown out or burned inside. The skin becomes so soft and glowing. It's a quick way to go towards the chakra system. Even though I learned the chakra system from Parshvanath, it is still a slow system until you put fuel on the fire. Even wrinkles will decrease if they happen prematurely.

Bones are the structure which hold the whole body. If they're full of toxins, your body will not be straight or as healthy as it can be. A healthy body is required first for meditation and chakra practices. You cannot really learn the chakra system then. It helps with alignment of the bones and straightening out the body. All the bones become detoxified. If someone has a hunchback it will help them a lot. I've helped many people with this problem and they got better completely.

If you're lacking white blood cells they will increase, and if you have enough, then they will become stronger. The white blood cells are our protective cells. We need them in the blood. Whenever you get a wound or a cut, all the white blood cells come to make a wall so the bacteria don't enter into your blood. They become very strong and the blood becomes purified. It will flow through your body in a balanced way. If you practice Purnam Yoga you won't have any chance of having blood clots or blocked arteries in the heart.

Each cell is toxic in us. We have millions of layers of toxins in our body. Millions of layers mean millions of cells. As soon as you start doing Purnam Yoga you will notice the clarity that you feel, and after 41 days you get the result of one or two layers of toxins beginning to burn up. Your vision will be stronger and you'll begin to feel the purpose of your life becoming clear. It takes 41 days for the toxins to burn, for one or two layers, that is the length of the cycle if you are really practicing. Hair doesn't have much purpose in our bodies, but when the channels are all cleared out it will help a person to be more positive, and they won't feel stress or be in bad thoughts that can cause their hair to fall out or break.

There are six senses in our body, but people are familiar only with five: touch, taste, smell, vision and hearing. Mind is the sixth sense. It doesn't have any structure, unlike the other five senses, but it is the king of the senses. All the senses will become so clear and active that you'll perceive the right thing. First, the nervous system is cleared, followed by the senses. The nervous system will send the messages to the senses, then to the brain, then the mind can grasp them, then the mind sends messages to the soul. All these things don't have their own intelligence, except the mind has a little bit only. All of them are like idiots, because whatever happens they have to take it. If you're hypnotized and touch something cold but it feels warm to you, your senses have no power to think for themselves. They are just feeling. Mind has a little intelligence but it's unsteady. When it's not steady, whatever message you get is sent to the soul, and the soul is the weakest of all of them. Whatever the nervous system gets, the senses, the brain and mind get, the soul has to get it. When your senses are clear, you'll perceive the right messages and truth, otherwise your body will keep you in illusion. Never mind what your goals are of reaching enlightenment, it doesn't matter if your body is not straightened out. It needs a lot of work. All these things are secretaries to the soul and they are complete idiots – they have no intelligence at all. Mind is always unsteady and doesn't care about anything. Just to drink, marry and enjoy. Nothing else. All the senses can be cleared, and when they are, they begin to get power and think.

Purnam Yoga can help clear the DNA of diabetes, and these kinds of diseases that you inherited; many incurable diseases. People just don't know how to get rid of them. They're in our DNA, and you can be at risk; even if you don't get it, it's there. DNA carries all kinds of stuff. Jains and Buddhists call it karma, but I call it toxins. Judaism and Catholicism call it sins, but they're talking about the same thing, because they disturb us. "Sin" comes from "toxins." That is the real meaning, and we can get rid of all of our toxins. They are not permanent if we make an effort. Our DNA is messed up; more than millions of layers in our DNA. The Purnam System will clear all these things in the body, then after the senses and mind, the toxins in our DNA are finally attacked. Even for just 20-30 minutes a day, after maybe three years the person will begin to see they have none of these diseases anymore if it's not too late for them to burn them. It will prevent these kinds of diseases, but if they're starting to become active and show on the surface, it will help decrease them. With stem-cell research, if we're successful, we can clear all the cells. Most of the diseases will disappear, but not all of them. DNA cannot be cleared that way, not all the way. Diabetes, for example, can be cleared out that way, but many other problems will not be affected by the stem-cell research.

All the toxins say good-bye to your body, but will take sometimes years and years. Maybe other toxins will be removed quickly, but on the deeper level it might take longer to clean the DNA. Until all the DNA is clear, you cannot get enlightened. Just to clean the toxins built up in the physical body from eating meat takes six years alone. And that is just the physical body, not the deeper things like the cells, the blood, or the subtle bodies. I am just talking about the organs, bones, tissues and muscles. Even if that much disappears you will be in a much better place and the toxins will move. They have no choice. They have to go because you are throwing them out.

If you're weak, you will become very strong. If you have sicknesses like migraines, they will disappear if you do the practice intensively. These kinds of problems, and problems with the senses and feelings of numbness will end after practicing Purnam Yoga. The toxins begin to move and the body becomes lighter and lighter. A lighter body has a better chance of having good blood circulation. Muscle pains, infections in the body – all of them will end. It will even happen quicker than antibiotics in some cases. If a person knows the system and they find symptoms of these things, they can prevent them from taking over their body.

Strength, flexibility and clearing your system out – this is what the Purnam System does for you. Yogis don't burn their karma, they burn their toxins. Once the toxins are burned the kundalini becomes active. Then you are going towards enlightenment when kundalini becomes active. Real yogis will work on their bodies first, because they know they cannot go further without it. They stay away from bad foods, sodas, alcohol, drugs, cigarettes, marijuana, all these things. They eat light foods, grains and fruits. For medicinal purposes, marijuana can help some people to deal with their pain, such as arthritis, but it doesn't reduce the actual root of the disease. It shouldn't be used for stress or entertainment, so do not fool yourself. When your body is clean and you put alcohol in your body it will get burned – hurt. If it's clean, like a baby's, give them a spoon of some Coca Cola and they will feel like something crazy is happening in their body. What about alcohol? Their body will get really hurt. Same thing, the yogi will never hurt their body. They stay away from those things.

The after-effects of practicing the Purnam System are beautiful. You sleep very well, you will begin eating well and you'll begin to want healthy foods. Your taste will change to enjoy those foods and your body will begin digesting much quicker. Your body will never feel heavy, it will always feel light, which will help you go deep into meditation.

Someone who has addictions, when they get into their practice of Purnam Yoga, what will happen is they will drop their addiction. The toxins that create the addiction are expelled from the body. It will help them to just drop the addiction right away. Drugs are very heavy on the body, and you don't want to be heavy anymore once you have experienced the feeling of a light body. It's like you're walking on earth but your footsteps feel so light and subtle to you, that it's as if you're not even

touching the ground. Alcohol, drugs and cigarettes make that heaviness. Marijuana is very addictive, even though many resist that truth. I've met people who were addicted to marijuana, claiming they are not addicted, but they get angry, agitated or upset if they miss one day. That's called an addiction. It might help someone with arthritis or other sickness to get through their pain, but not in a permanent way. They have to smoke every day to only get a few hours of relief. It doesn't get rid of the problem. Any addiction is not good, no matter what it is. Addiction brings karma to you.

It's not difficult to learn the Purnam System. Children are even able to do it and they do. We teach them at our Spiritual Children's Camp (SpiritualChildrensCamp.com). You will feel some dizziness during a good practice, and you can rest for a few days if it seems like a lot to you. Sometimes a certain type of body cannot take intensive breathing and they might feel some discomfort for a few days, but it is normal for that kind of body. All the emotions will come on the surface and attack you when you practice Purnam yoga. You might cry, jealousy might come on the way, hate, negativity, or you will suffer through your emotions – all kinds of emotions. They will come up because the body is now getting clear, and all these emotions are built up in the toxins in you. When the body is full of toxins, the emotions will not affect the body much, but when you start to clear them out, the emotions are able to touch you more deeply. Eventually, though, when it's clear and more balanced, the emotions will not bring you up and down anymore.

Step by step, if you do it intensively, Purnam Yoga will clear all the toxins out of you. Toxins block everything. As long as you follow this system slowly, which is what we teach at Siddhayatan, you're not far away from enlightenment. It will take time, but you're taking the steps to get there. First, clean your body and follow nonviolence. It won't happen suddenly. If you ate meat in your past lives those toxins carry into your next lives through your DNA. All of these need to go. Any weak thing needs an instrument, and the soul is weak. It needs the body. Soul is wandering in the dark all the time and doesn't have the sense to wake up. It's asleep like someone under the influence of drugs all the time. If the instrument is dirty or heavy, you cannot use it properly. If your glasses are dirty can you see through them? It's the same idea.

Ashtanga yoga is merely exercise for the body. Postures are a very slow system to make you healthy and detoxified. Purnam Yoga is very quick in comparison. It affects you after a few days, where postures may take months to have any real effect. Ashtanga means eight-limbed, the eight steps of yoga. Though if you go to an Ashtanga yoga class, they teach you only the asanas, postures. So, why do they call it Ashtanga? They're supposed to teach all the steps, but they're learning merely postures. Whoever gave the name was wrong. People go to the gym and they feel better, right? They exercise the body, run a little bit and their blood circulation changes. Same thing if you do asanas, it's going to help you in the long run. You have to be dedicated. Ashtanga is the whole system, the eight steps, and I have come across many people who claim to practice the steps, but they still drink or do drugs and even eat meat and eggs. They just jump to the third step, and it's wrong. They don't get any benefit from their practice without following the disciplines first. With Purnam Yoga, you do 41 days of practice and keep from eating meat or drinking alcohol, then see how you feel. What they teach in popular yoga styles are difficult postures. It makes your physical body healthy in the long run, but it doesn't burn the toxins, the karma. If you follow only one limb, the postures, it's not enough. Hatha yoga is the same. Many people teaching Hatha yoga recommend the disciplines, but in Ashtanga places they don't teach them usually. They have no idea what they are. How will they reach enlightenment or samadhi?

There is a story: one Muslim guy, he was always drunk. He spent all his money on drinking, until he had to sell all of his things to buy more alcohol. His family became very poor. They lost all their money and their house – all their things gone. This guy started going to his friends and others to borrow money, and after a while they became scared. After he kept repeatedly asking, they started to refuse him, and he couldn't find anyone. So, he walked into a mosque, and he found the imam, the priest.

"Look, I am very happy that I came to your temple here. I want to see some kind of miracle."

"What kind of miracle do you want to see?" the imam replied to this drunk guy.

"Can you make this mosque move?"

"Of course not. I am not God, I am just a priest."

The man was disappointed. "How long have you been a priest?" he asked.

"I've been a priest for 45 years."

"Wow... 45 years a priest, and you cannot even make this mosque move? Give me a little bit of alcohol and you'll see how fast it spins!"

Those people who are doing Ashtanga or Hatha yoga, they have no idea they're supposed to follow the nonviolent system of discipline first. They are merely doing exercise.

You have the instrument, the super-instrument. If you want to realize what God is, if you want to be liberated from all your suffering, it's not out of your reach. Use your instrument properly. You got it because of your karma. Now start cleaning it and working on it. It is going to wake up the soul slowly.

Appa so paramappa; your soul is the *paramappa*, the absolute soul. *Appa* means your self, your soul, and paramappa means God. Basically, soul is the seed and paramatma is the tree. So, if this soul becomes a tree one day, that is paramatma. It's very simple. You are God. Paramappa and paramatma mean the same thing.

I always tell people that if you know mathematics or science, I have a very simple formula. Your soul is surrounded by matter. *Atma* is soul, and *prakriti* is matter, coming from Sanskrit. Matter means particles; all the particles in the universe and they're always surrounding us. When something has particles you're able to see it. Even karma is matter, but you have to be in a higher state of consciousness to see it. So, all things that are visible in the universe are called "matter." When you have atma, and combine it with prakriti, it becomes *jivatma*, a living being. Where there is soul in the grip of matter, it's called jivatma, because it has a body. Karma creates the body. The formula is:

Soul (atma), plus matter (prakriti), equals a living being (jivatma). Once you understand this formula, it's very easy to reverse it:

A living being (jivatma), minus matter (prakriti), equals God (paramatma).

The living being without all the matter, all the karma and particles, becomes the absolute soul, God. That is moksha, or liberation, when you become the absolute soul, Siddha. Karma creates the body, so if a person can burn all their karmas through spiritual practices and discipline, they will not get another body. They are freed from the cycle of birth and death. All the liberated souls make up God, just as all the drops of water make up the ocean. That is why we say, "appa so paramappa," soul is God. All the people who think that enlightened masters return to Earth are in illusion. If someone merges with God, they become that; they have no karmas left, and karma is what takes you from life to life, body to body. If Jesus merged with God, he cannot come back. Same thing with Mahavira, or Buddha, Krishna, or any other person. When you become Siddha, you remain Siddha. Siddha is body-less.

The body is matter. Soul has no matter, it is just in the grip of matter, but not touched by it. Any substance is made out of particles. The particles here, the light, the room you're in is full of particles. If you have seen it, when the sunlight will come through a window and light up all the dust and you can see it floating around, it is like that. But the particles are even more subtle that you cannot even see them with the naked eyes. The dust you see is physical matter, but not yet subtle. This whole universe is full of the subtlest matter. As soon as we think negative, those particles automatically come towards us. We are inviting them. It builds and becomes layers upon layers, darker and darker, until one day it will block your light fully. You don't have to go somewhere else to collect matter. They are around you already. They don't even come to you, even though they surround you, unless you invite them. You get angry, they come to you suddenly. It's so automatic. As soon as you think negative, they will just come towards you and they make one more layer, another layer and another layer. So, soul is in the grip of millions of millions of layers of karma. Guess who is inviting them? Appa. You are. Without invitation they don't bother you; they're like the American police. American police will not bother you at all if you don't break the rules. Right? Indian police will bother you. If you're driving your car without your license, but you're not breaking any rules on the road, then the police won't bother you. As long as your car is registered, insured, they will not bother you. But if you make a mistake they will come to you. In the same way, if you don't invite these particles that are floating everywhere, they will not come to you. Become greedy, you're inviting them. Become a stealer, killer, hater, you're inviting them. Any time you're angry or upset, you're inviting them.

But who invites them 24 hours a day? People who are like the Klu Klux Klan. Because they're full of hate, full of anger and prejudice. Even if you invite these particles one time, it makes a big layer around you. What about those people who are negative for 24 hours a day? All the time in their anger? Even in their dreams they are in that state, and they invite them there, too. They just indulge in ignorance all the time. They don't know what they're doing. Maybe some of their layers of karma can be removed if you give them a chance, but sometimes the Nikachita karma is too much that they can't be helped. I can give many examples in my life. I gave a lot of people chances. Even people who tell me that they were in jail, or doing bad things, got in some accidents, or similar situations, I would still give them a chance. Sometimes they get the help, but they cannot receive it. The Nikachita karmas are in the way and they cannot be helped. Why? Because the layers are so dense you cannot even penetrate any particles of help. It's very difficult. Sometimes even if God comes in front of you, you cannot be helped. That is called Nikachita karma. Nobody can break it, not even God.

But there are other things. Maybe they're not Nikachita karmas, but another kind of karma and they have many layers surrounding them. They can be penetrated and they suddenly wake up. It happens rarely, but it's possible. It's not that they don't have a lot of karma to work on, they just maybe didn't collect certain ones that prevent them. Nikachita karma you have to go through, but others you can break without going through them. It's difficult sometimes; you want help, but because of your karma you cannot be helped, even by an enlightened master. Their karma needs to be lessened a little bit before the help can get through. Somehow their path is blocked. It happens all the time with many people. If you prevent others from doing good, you will be blocked from receiving good.

It can happen the other way around, too. They can get help right away, they're suddenly awake. There is a Buddhist teaching, a saying: some people are so asleep that you have to literally throw a bucket of water on them to wake them up. If they wake up, that is fortunate, but there are three other kinds of sleepers. You shake them, and maybe they will wake up. Another kind who sleeps a little lighter, you just go there and touch them, not even shaking, and they wake up. Sometimes you can just call their name and they suddenly wake up. It can happen this way.

Let me share with you a story about an Indian man who became a swami. A mother was waking up her son, and his name was Gopal.

"Gopal, wake up, wake up. Gopal, wake up! The sun has risen, it's a beautiful morning, the dark has disappeared. Night has gone. How long will you sleep Gopal?"

Children change their sides when they don't want to get up, and he rolled over and slept some more. His mother started cooking his lunch to take to school, and his books are ready.

"Gopal, wake up!"

Suddenly a man was passing by on the street and he heard this. His name was Gopal, too. He stopped. He used to go on a morning walk every day. He heard it again.

"Gopal, how long will you sleep, Gopal? The sun has risen, it's a beautiful morning, the dark has disappeared. Night has gone."

The more she said it, the more it hit his heart deeply. He forgot about his morning walk and went back to his home. He told his wife to wake everyone up. He asked his sons to bring his bags. They asked what happened, and he repeated,

"The sun has risen..." he repeated what he heard on the street. His children thought he went crazy. He told them they wouldn't understand. He repeated it again and again. This man later became a very popular swami in India.

You have to go deep inside and understand the real meaning of things. The problem is all the toxins in your body, all of your karmas, they prevent you from seeing clearly. Even you think you see clearly, you are living with those toxins like the fisherman living with the smell of fish. You don't notice what is wrong because it has always been with you.

After just one hour of Purnam Yoga your aura changes a lot. Ashtanga and Hatha yoga don't affect you in this way. The aura becomes bright and it shows that toxins are being removed right away. It is very intensive. It makes you full of energy. You'll even be able to work for 15 hours a day and you won't feel tired at all; it creates tremendous energy in you. All the channels are clear. Your body becomes very light, and a light body cannot stay asleep like a heavy body. Some people sleep for 10 hours, 12 hours even. Half the day is finished before they even get out of bed. The heavy body cannot get deep rest because of the toxins and foods don't digest. All of your nadis will become balanced. The Ida, Pingala and Sushumna will be balanced with each other, and breath will flow equally. The Sushumna is the symbol of kundalini, and Purnam Yoga helps you to jump into the shushumna quicker, because you burn the things blocking your way. Any time you are positive, feeling light, eating healthy, your energy will flow upward. Kundalini will begin to flow upward.

I personally invite you to take our Purnam Yoga retreat at Siddhayatan if you want to get these benefits. You can learn more at http://siddhayatan.org/yogaretreat.

PRANAYAMA

In the yogic system there is a very important technique called pranayama, or controlled breathing, as most people translate it. You have to breathe in a certain way to receive the benefits. Yogis use the word nadi; these are the main nerves where breath flows through the body. Some people might describe a sensation or imagery of breath going down the spine to the tailbone. The breath can feel like it is going down the center of the spine, or down the right side, or down the left side, or possibly spiraling around like the picture which Western doctors use of two snakes coiled around a pole: the Caduceus, or kundalini symbol, the double helix. Remember, when you breathe in a balanced way, you automatically breathe through the Sushumna nadi. This feels like the air is going straight down through the middle of the spine. Only a healthy person or a baby, or a yogi, can breathe through the Sushumna nadi. You can call this effortless breathing. If your nadis are working properly, it means you are in touch with your original center, the navel.

You have to understand that breathing through the Sushumna nadi is not a special yogic technique that must be learned. It comes naturally and doesn't require effort. When a person is feeling normal, not in any tension at all, he or she will automatically breathe through the Sushumna. If a person is natural and relaxed, they cannot be angry, or proud, or violent, or greedy. Not even if they were being crucified like Jesus, or being made to drink poison, like Socrates. Or even being stoned, or having sharp nails pushed into their ears as Mahavira. That is the real relaxation. It happens when your breathing switches to the Sushumna and you can be very still and silent inside. Once you are in the Sushumna nadi you have everything: peace, stillness, compassion and joy. Because people eat without much regard for the actual content of the food, they take many impurities into their stomach and intestines. This causes blockages in the nervous system and in the nadis, which you can clear by breathing exercises. In the Purnam System, these breathing techniques are combined with postures to create an intense heat inside of you, the fire that can burn the toxins. There are several methods for controlling which nostril the breath is coming through.

Press your finger or thumb against the outside of the nostril to close it. Start by using your right ring finger against the left side of your nose, to close the left nostril. Breathe in through the right nostril. Hold your breath inside for a moment, while you release your finger at the same time from your left nostril and use your thumb to close your right nostril. Now breathe out through the left nostril.

When your nervous system and nadis have been completely cleaned by this method, then you automatically begin breathing through the Sushumna. Then it is impossible to be angry or jealous or greedy. Mahavira, Buddha and Jesus were always breathing through their Sushumna. That is why they did not get angry or have any of the negative attitudes of common people such as violence or pride. The Sushumna comes very close to your original center, so in India all yogis emphasize the Sushumna nadi. By doing these practices, you will automatically connect to your main center again. You'll be in love always, you'll feel oneness with every living being. Only then you will find your real individual role in this universe. Be aware of your actions, words and habits.

Breathing is important for each chakra, because the breath is fire. When you breathe correctly, the fire works in your body. If you know how to breathe, you will know how to be healthy and your chakras will be balanced. I say the breath is fire because when you take a breath in a certain way, inside of you fire is created. Suppose you inhale through your Pingala nadi, it can create a lot of heat inside of your body and your digestive system will work very well. It burns everything, all the negative stuff, bad bacteria. The breath is burning, but you have to know the right system, the right way to do pranayama. "Ayama" means you control the prana, it's under your control. It means your system begins to cooperate with you when you go through all the system and clean your whole body and mind.

Prana is our life-force and it doesn't go out of control when it cooperates with you. The breath always stays balanced, natural and relaxed, like a baby. That is the real meaning of pranayama – when the breath is fully balanced. People misinterpret the meaning of it, that you have to force yourself and control your breath. That will only create tension. Tension blocks meditation. Many people recommend that you should control the length of each breath by counting numbers. They say to inhale for eight seconds, suppose, then hold it for four seconds, and finally exhale for ten seconds. The important thing is for the breath to follow your own natural rhythm, not an artificial system. Except in sleep or deep meditation, then it will flow differently by itself. If counting is helpful, that's okay, but it is better to let your breath come naturally. Breathe when you want to breathe. When a person is in a truly relaxed state, they can feel when their lungs want a new breath of air, so immediately they take a breath in. The lungs get full and they slow down. If the lungs want to rest, they might pause between their breaths. When you breathe this way, according to your own body, you might notice the lungs have an appetite for breathing. Ordinarily we don't feel this desire unless something unusual is happening, like when our air supply is cut off somehow, or by counting numbers and holding our breath when the lungs desire to have another breath. Singers feel this when they have a longer note to complete before they can have another breath of air.

Natural breathing, breathing according to our lungs' desire, is one of the greatest physical pleasures for a human. There are two reasons. The first is that air is our most important physical need, so the desire for air is always the strongest sensation we feel. Hunger and thirst are immediately forgotten if our air supply is interrupted. You can have a big feast in front of you, but what can your body do with the food if there is no air to breathe? Even physical pain can be forgotten, like when someone is burning in a house, they will go through all the flames just to breathe air. When the desire for air is noticed, all other sensations are forgotten right away. It's like a safety feature built into our nervous system. The second reason is because the desire for air is the only desire that can always be fulfilled exactly on time. As soon as you have the desire, you can fulfill it right away. With other desires, there is always some delay. If you feel hungry, you might have to cook first, or go and buy something to eat. If you feel sleepy, you have to change out of your clothes, or go home. Even if a glass of water is sitting on the table in front of you, you have to decide to pick it up, and bring it to your mouth. Only the air for your next breath is always ready; no waiting at all. So, even if you cannot distinguish which nadi your breath is using, if you begin to breathe more by your own natural timing, by your lungs' desire, it will give you so much benefit. It will eventually bring you into the Sushumna nadi.

Why don't we normally feel this desire and the pleasure of taking each breath? It's very simple. Since we were babies, we have been taught not to feel it. The same thing has happened to our natural hunger and thirst. Remember when you were very little, if you were playing a game outdoors, you would play for hours and hours and forget about eating. Suddenly your body becomes so hungry and you stop playing immediately to go and eat. That is what it means to eat naturally, when your body feels it, and it is a great pleasure. Even if the food is very plain. Normally we are taught not to let our hunger increase to this point. Long before a child feels any hunger, their parents ask them to come for dinner, or maybe try to tempt them with sweets. We form the habit of such frequent meals and snacks that real hunger cannot occur.

In the same way, we develop the habit of unnatural breathing, which spoils the appetite for deep, natural breaths. We learn these habits from our families and society. Grandparents will tease a baby, tickle them, and try to force a laugh out of them and interrupt their breathing. They want to have the baby's attention, and the baby will start to acclimate to their way of breathing even. Just as the baby is tempted by sweets and other things, they are tempted with artificial laughter and excitement as well. Soon they become dependent on another's company, and in many cases, their approval. When the child has learned to breathe in time with their grandparents and parents, then when they misbehave, all the parents have to do is slow their breathing down and have a serious expression, and immediately the baby becomes ashamed or worried. It is easier for the babies to cry or stop their game, do whatever the parents want, than just breathe by themselves. We were taught not to breathe naturally, from the navel.

A person who is following his own desire to breathe, according to the pace set by the chemistry of their body, they cannot be emotionally manipulated at all. Only after a child's center has moved up from the navel to the chest can they be emotionally controlled. When you can move your own breathing back to your abdomen, no one will be able to affect you by playing with your emotions. Your aura will be full of love and good energy always. Whether you are alone or if people are abusing you, you can still breathe freely.

For the first chakra, Muladhara, you need to practice the *Surya Bhedi pranayama*. The right nostril is open, the Pingala, or sun channel. Close your left nostril, the moon channel, with your ring finger. Breathe in deeply through your right nostril. Your breath needs to be steady, deep and not quick. Don't rush. When you can't bring in any more air, close your right nostril by pressing your thumb down against the side of your nose, and exhale in the same manner, steady and relaxed, through your left nostril, through the Ida nadi. Now that you've exhaled through your left nostril, close it once again and repeat the steps, inhaling through your Pingala nadi. In between breaths, hold the air inside of you, count to maybe ten or fifteen seconds. Then you exhale. If there is no energy in the first chakra, there is no current or force. By bringing air into your system through your Pingala nadi, you are building up heat, and when you exhale through your Ida nadi, you are pushing the cool air out of your body. After 50 or 60 cycles of this you build up so much heat in your body that you'll become very warm, and maybe even begin to sweat.

The Muladhara needs a lot of heat to open up. Its color is red, like fire. Surya Bhedi pranayama will activate it automatically, and if you keep up with your practice of this technique it will get stronger and stronger. Plus, you won't be cold anymore.

Your second chakra, *Svadhisthana*, needs cool air to help balance it. It is just the opposite of the Muladhara chakra. Cool air is created by practicing *Chandra Bhedi pranayama*. It is the same technique as Surya Bhedi pranayama, but you switch the nostrils you are inhaling and exhaling through. Surya Bhedi creates heat, because you pull air in through your surya nadi, and Chandra Bhedi creates coolness, because the air is being inhaled through your Ida nadi.

Begin by closing your right nostril with your thumb. Slowly inhale through your left nostril, and when you can't breathe in any longer, hold your breath for ten to fifteen seconds. While you hold your breath in, release your thumb from your right nostril and close your left nostril with your ring finger. Now you can slowly exhale through your right nostril to push the warm air out. If you have a lot of heat in your body, especially for women who are going through menopause and have hot-flashes, this pranayama will not only balance the second chakra but reduce the intense heat in the body. It will help you to stay calm and feel balanced. When you practice a lot and your Svadhisthana chakra begins to balance, you will feel like you've come back home and you can relax.

The third chakra, Manipura, is near the navel and needs to be hit very hard. Not like somebody hitting you, it needs to be shocked, and you need a lot of oxygen in your blood. *Kapalbhati pranayama* will hit your navel this way. Keep your mouth closed for this pranayama. You breathe only through your nostrils and it will be very intensive.

Start by taking a normal breath, not too deep, and then you suddenly pull your entire abdomen in towards your stomach like you're trying to squeeze it very hard. It's not a long motion, it happens very quickly, very suddenly. You pull your abdomen in very fast and it will make you exhale with a lot of force through your nostrils. There will be a big sound when you exhale, because it's like blowing your nose. You want to do it with a lot of force. As soon as you exhale through your nostrils, you relax your abdomen and automatically you'll inhale more air, then right away you repeat it again.

When you practice Kapalbhati pranayama you'll feel a lot of heat and you will feel dizzy when you practice it intensely. The Manipura chakra balances out when it is activated, and you won't get any discomforting feelings or be affected by any criticism.

Practicing baby breathing, *Baal Rechanvidhi pranayama*, will also help the Manipura. Inhale slowly through your nostrils, deeply, but use your diaphragm to pull in the oxygen and not your chest. Hold the breath for five to seven seconds and then exhale slowly, but naturally. Repeat again. Your stomach becomes like a balloon when you inhale, and it shrinks very small when you exhale, because you squeeze the air out.

The *Anaahat* chakra is the fourth chakra, and it needs a lot of oxygen as well. Practice *Anulom Vilom pranayama* to help open the Anaahat chakra. Always begin from the right nostril when practicing Anulom Vilom. With your right ring finger, close your left nostril and inhale slowly through your Pingala nadi, the right nostril. When you reach the most that you can inhale, switch your nostrils by closing the right and opening the left, and now exhale through your Ida nadi, the left nostril. Keep your fingers remaining where they are to now inhale through your Ida nadi. When you can't inhale anymore breath, switch your nostrils again so the left is closed once more, and the right is open. Exhale through your right nostril. This is one cycle of Anulom Vilom pranayama. It brings a lot of oxygen, and the element of the Anaahat chakra is air. All of your emotions will begin to balance out and affect you less and less. It brings a lot of oxygen into your body and your blood, because it's a slow practice. When it's more slow it brings a lot if it's done right. This will clear the main nadis and help your blood a lot.

There is another pranayama, *Urdhavrechan pranayama*, which will open the heart. It's not mentioned anywhere because no one knows about it. People are in illusion that the *Yoga Sutras* hold everything. First, place your tongue behind your teeth, pressing very lightly on the back of the bottom row. Make your lips pursed like a small "O," and slowly inhale. It will feel cold and maybe icy. When you can't bring anymore air into your lungs, hold your breath and look up to the ceiling with your eyes wide open. Then, breathe out forcefully through your nostrils 50 times, similar to the Kapalbhati technique. Then lower your head back to center and repeat the breathing exercise again.

Vishuddhi, the fifth chakra, will be affected by *Nadi Shodhan pranayama*. Close your left nostril with your right ring finger, and push out your breath forcefully on the right side, twice. It's like Kapalbhati pranayama, because of the intensity, but only one nostril at a time is open. The inhalation will happen naturally when your abdomen is released, so try not to think about it too much. On each side you have to exhale twice before switching to the opposite nostril. Keep your mouth closed. So, close your left nostril and forcefully push all your breath out through your right nostril two times. It has to be very quick and with intensity. Now switch to open your left nostril and close your right nostril and repeat again, exhaling twice through your left nostril. That is one cycle of nadi shodhan – twice through each nostril. This will clear your throat chakra, and it helps the thyroid gland to produce normal acidity. Saliva will balance out and food will be digested the right way. Try to start by practicing 10 cycles – 20 exhalations – on each nostril, a day. If the nadis are not clear you won't be able to talk clearly, even if you're a scholar.

Shanmukhi Mudra pranayama is for the sixth chakra, the *Ajna* chakra. It clears all the senses. Start by pursing your lips tightly and placing the tip of your tongue on the back of your lower teeth. Inhale a long breath through your lips. It will feel tight, as if you're breathing through a straw, and make a sound like the wind, with a cool sensation on your tongue. Take in as much breath as you can, and when you are about to finish your inhalation, bring both of your hands up near your head. It will take some practice to do it the right way, because as soon as you finish your inhalation you need to close your senses with your hands. When you cannot inhale more, place your thumbs pressing in your ears to close them, place your ring and pinky fingers across your lips to stop air from coming out, place your middle fingers on your nostrils to shut them, and your index fingers to keep both of your eyelids shut. This is the way you prevent air from moving in and out. As soon as your fingers are in place, begin trying to push all your breath out. It has nowhere to go, so your cheeks will expand like a balloon, and you'll feel tension in your head from the pressure. Hold as long as you can, and when you're ready to let it go, release your hands right away and let the breath exhale out of you as fast as it needs to. Don't try to push it, just let it be natural.

Do this process for three to five times; it will clear your senses out and open the Ajna chakra, the third-eye. It's like an exercise for your mind and your brain. Shan means "six;" including your mind, that is the six senses. When you feel light-headed you suddenly go into the sixth chakra and begin to think positively.

For the *Sahasrara* chakra, the seventh chakra, you need to be sitting to practice this pranayama. It is called *Adhorechan pranayama*. Place both of your hands on your knees, and bending from your tailbone, go all the way down with your whole torso, like you are going to touch the ground in front of you with your chin. Don't bend or compress the stomach. As you come up, slowly inhale and bring your torso back to the straight position. When you reach the peak of your inhalation and your back is fully straight, now you forcefully exhale all of the air through your nose by pulling in your abdomen tightly and quickly throwing your torso back down so your face comes close to the ground again, but it has to be quick, it has to happen in one motion. The forceful exhalation and throwing your torso forward has to be in one quick motion.

This pranayama will clear your entire head. Do it 50 times at least. Don't worry if you feel dizzy, because you are clearing a lot of things in your head, the glands in your brain, too, so it's normal to feel dizzy. It shows the toxins are moving. After a while you'll begin to see hundreds of thousands of stars in front of you. Adhorechan pranayama is not mentioned in any yogic texts because the people who wrote them didn't know the real system. Your seventh chakra will open. This is coming from the Purnam System that I created almost 150 years ago; it is very powerful.

By practicing pranayama techniques, doing the intensive breathing, your nadis will be cleared and the right messages can be carried throughout your system. Nervous system, blood, all channels will be cleared and the body will be cleared. You move towards spirituality when your body is clear. The colors in your aura become brighter and radiate more; it indicates the person is moving more to spirituality. Millions of layers of toxins are inside you and they begin to burn. It is beautiful; you begin to see the clear vision and have clarity, the true vision. Otherwise you just flow in the worldly thinking, worries and desires, not trying to find the higher things.

You have to be careful when you practice pranayama though. I will say not to overdo it. When a person over-does their pranayama practice, their body can become very fat. They can become like Swami Muktananda's guru. It's better just to do one or two hours. It won't bother you, but if you do too much, any more than that, you lose control over your body. When you're overdoing it, instead of burning the toxins it brings something different and changes your system. It's like when you fast but you drink too much water, you will gain weight. Even though you're not eating any food for days, you still gain weight.

Also, if you do these intensive breathing exercises too much and too fast, you can become very negative – the opposite result you are seeking. This happens because your body and brain cannot handle the quick detoxification process. I warned several students not to do thousands of repetitions of their pranayama, and they did not listen. They became extremely negative and went faraway from their goals. So be careful to not over-do your practices.

Never do pranayama before you go to sleep. At night, the trees reverse their processes and produce a lot of carbon dioxide. Instead of breathing in very pure oxygen like in the early morning just before sunrise, you're inhaling carbon dioxide. With the intensity of pranayama, you flood your system with carbon dioxide. The best time to practice is during the morning, beginning 90 minutes before the sun rises. All the trees at this time start producing tremendous oxygen until the sun rises, and throughout the day it turns slowly to carbon dioxide. It's better not to practice pranayama after sunset. There is less oxygen later in the day than earlier in the morning. People are also mostly asleep before the sun rises, and when everyone is asleep there is no chaos. Otherwise, when they wake up they turn on the T.V., and they watch negative news. When so many people do this, it creates negative energy all over. The thoughts go downward in that negativity, and thoughts are moving. Unless you're in a higher state, it will disturb you if you try to meditate at this time.

That's why we call it *Brahma muhurta*, the Godly time, because negativities are minimized. At night they are not minimized. Even at midnight, people are still up eating, drinking, doing negative things. Early morning is quiet and people are asleep. "Brahma" means "God," and "muhurta" means "time." Godly time. Oxygen is very important. The trees

reverse and create tremendous oxygen during this time. It helps to stay healthy and plus it's a quiet time so you can go into deep meditation.

Have control with your practice and be patient and steady. Depending on your spiritual practices, start by just doing 30 minutes in the morning, altogether. Increase slowly, 2 to 5 minutes every couple days. One hour is enough to get good effects, but if you want to do more, up to two hours won't harm you if you have the time. Your mind will be really light and it won't disturb you any longer.

You will learn the breathing techniques for each chakra when I go into detail later, this way you can help them become more balanced and return to your center. The breathing exercises among other chakra awakening techniques can be viewed at: http://chakraawakeningbook.com/suite this way you do them properly. It will work if you practice. You have to be consistent and dedicated. All your emotions and energy will be straightened out, and you will become very natural. When you start reading about the chakras, you will have everything that you need to get started.

MANTRA: THE DIVINE SOUND

All the different yoga postures improve your health, because all of them in some way help the navel area. If your navel is working properly, then you do not feel like hating others or killing or harming any other creature. The fact that civilized people are mostly disconnected from the navel center is what causes them to get mentally disturbed, always having the feelings of insecurity, jealousy, anger, and going up and down in their emotions. Chanting mantras will also help you to reunite with your navel center. Chant loudly, and make the sounds come from the navel. When you are really connected with your center you will have all the good qualities like love, nonviolence, compassion, sympathy, truth, non-stealing, and harmony with every living being.

Mantra means "divine sound." It can purify you by cleaning the heart of all negativities and tensions. Repeating a mantra can clear your system of all its impurities. It will then also protect you in the future from any further negative vibrations affecting your soul. There are both good and bad sounds in the universe. Sounds are not just letters of the alphabet. In every language the scholars tell us that the spoken words came first. Only much later did people create a system of written letters to record the sounds that were already being spoken. So, written letters are less natural, more artificial. But speech itself is eternal. Its sounds are natural; they come from inside of you.

It is important to always create good sounds, divine sounds. All good sounds have a positive result right away. It's just the opposite with bad sounds. We attract the negative particles of karma and not only will our soul be in even more darkness, but our energy goes down as well. If you say a bad word, a word that can hurt somebody, you have that negativity in you right away. When you use these words to abuse someone, or even simply name-calling, the person will have a negative reaction. But if you praise someone, or say sweet things, the person has a positive reaction. One makes you angry or upset, and one makes you peaceful. It makes that vibration in you and you feel it through your emotions. Bad sounds include profanity, negative words and abusive language. Such sounds create negative vibrations and attract impurities, causing a bad environment. That is why it is very important to pay attention to what kind of sounds you are making, because you will get the results of them whether you like it or not, regardless of if you want them or not.

The meaning of mantra is, the purest sound that creates the highest vibration. The sounds are combined in a way that makes electricity, and that electricity can purify you. Wherever it vibrates in you, it purifies. Electricity goes out when you recite the mantra and it purifies the air and enters back into your body.

In Eastern cultures and philosophies there is one very popular mantra: *aum*. Aum represents the name of God. It is a very simple and natural sound that is easy for anyone to pronounce. According to Hindu culture, we can break down aum as follows:

A – stands for Brahma, the creative power of God

U – stands for Vishnu, the sustaining power of God

M – stands for Shiva, the destructive power of God

The actual meaning of these three aspects of God – creating, sustaining and destroying – are not as important as the vibration that aum creates in you. When you chant aum, it creates a vibration that strongly affects your body and your soul. Unfortunately, many Hindus believe Brahma, Vishnu, and Shiva to be God. That is not true, they are simply powers.

As I said, aum is a divine sound and a natural sound. In fact, it is the first sound uttered by a newborn. If you're observant and pay close attention, you'll find that the first sound he makes is "A... a... a..." This is why in every language the first letter of the alphabet is "A."

The second sound the baby makes is "U." At first the baby is fed from the mother's breast. Then it is necessary for them to learn to eat other food in order to live. When they miss the taste of their mother's milk they cry, "U... u... u..."

After a little while the baby begins to get more control over the opening and closing movement of their lips, and they begin to make a totally new sound: "M... m... m..." They are cooing because this sound is easy and natural for the baby to make. This is why aum is a natural sound. Remember that only natural things belong to God. The more unnatural or artificial you are, the further you will be from soul.

Many people do not know how to make the natural divine sound aum. It is very important that this sound should be made from your center, the navel. Any sound that originates from the navel will sound natural and sweet. To speak from your throat or chest is unnatural. When you speak from the chest it means you are trying to make your voice sound sweet, but this will not produce an effective positive vibration. Just speak naturally, don't make any effort when you speak. Be natural and nature will help you. If a person does not have a sweet voice but practices singing from the navel, the original center, then one day he or she will sing very well. It is only a matter of practicing. Their voice will become attractive and sweet. It takes time but it can be achieved.

Mantras have existed since millions of years ago. They are not created, because all the sounds are already there. Sound is around us all the time. It is just a matter of knowing the sounds and how they work. It is possible for anyone to create a mantra by putting these sounds together, but there is one condition, though: the person has to have absolute perfection in *Matrikavidya*, the system of how sounds work together. It is an ancient system, and no one really knows it anymore. When you put sounds together it will create a certain color, aura and electricity. If a person is well-versed in that kind of knowledge then they can put together a mantra. It's not that they create it. All sounds exist already, they just learn how they go together. You don't have to be enlightened. An enlightened master just knows the sounds already, so it is natural for them. When you say, "Aa" what does it create? Is it fire? Coolness? What colors does it make? You have to have the perfect knowledge in that system. The sound creates the certain kind of light around you and it protects you if you have strength in the mantra, if you are always reciting it consistently. When you even just think about it, even without reciting it, it protects you. You need that strength, so always learn the good mantras and practice them all the time. After some time the power begins to come to you, even if you don't want it. The meaning of the mantra is "*Mananat trayate iti mantra;*" when you recite a mantra, it protects you.

Mantras have to be recited in the Prakrit and Sanskrit languages, very old languages, which have very strong vibrations in their sounds. That is how the sounds work. No other languages have this kind of power in their alphabet. Suppose that you want a mantra in German or Spanish or some other language, you can get a phrase, but not a mantra. New Age people have created "Aum Namaha Christaya," or "I bow to Christ." You cannot make up words and call it a mantra. The other languages were not made with those higher vibrations in the sounds. They were lost after a long time and the modern languages don't have it anymore. First of all, mantra is a word coming from Prakrit, which became Sanskrit later on. If other languages don't have this word "mantra," then they don't have the understanding of what it is. They have their own alphabetic words, but no mantras.

Prayers can be in any language, because when you're doing a prayer you're in positive thoughts and trying to focus on something higher. But the mantra is not a prayer. When you really recite a mantra, you're not asking, you're just doing. You are just in the sound fully, and that is when you get the results. You feel the electricity in you and you feel your body lighten and your mind calms down. A prayer can help you in that direction if you are really into it, but it doesn't have the same effect. So the mantras have to be in those two languages.

In Adinath's time, language was not developed enough, so there was little communication through language, compared to today. It began slowly, but it was enough for people to understand each other. We call it *Boli*, it means you just understand. Before there was a written system, people who spoke only were called Boli – no rules or grammar and structures. Whether you spoke like a child or an adult, as long as you could understand, it didn't matter. Prakrit in the very beginning is not even the same Prakrit we can understand today, which is still ancient. If you don't put much grammar into language, it will survive much longer. Once you make grammar, it becomes structured and the language dissolves faster because of the way societies change. American English will survive longer than British English, because it has flexibility. In America, nobody cares what you sound like as long as you can be understood. This is why Prakrit survived through everything, even though very few people know it now. Many other languages just disappear.

Sanskrit means reformed. It's a language reformed from Prakrit. Panini was the first grammarian who made the rules and structure for it, and Sanskrit has a lot of structure. It's very difficult to learn, you have to memorize many different rules. Sanskrit is no more than 4,000 years old, maximum. You can say between 3,000 and 4,000 years old. It started in what is now known as Kabul, Afghanistan. India used to be such a big country. Cambodia used to be part of India. That's why everywhere in Cambodia you find Vishnu temples and Buddhist temples, ruins thousands of years old. Before 4,000 years, there were less rules and it was closer to Prakrit, but the real reformed Sanskrit started around that time. Even the Vedas are not written in real Sanskrit, but we call it Sanskrit. Sanskrit died because they made too much structure in it, too many rules. It's considered a dead language except for in scriptures.

When you recite a mantra, even if there are people sitting near and not reciting anything, they will feel the vibration, too. Mantras are very strong. They'll feel something in their body, heat or warmth or a little vibration. Sound is eternal. Once it's recited, it will travel from one galaxy to another and it keeps going. Wherever it's reaching, it creates that electricity there and the whole universe is affected by it. That is why it is very important to watch your speech!

Sounds cannot be blocked from anywhere; it travels all over. It's slow, but it travels, and wherever it goes you can catch it. You need the right instrument. If I speak today, after a thousand years this sound might travel to the stars outside this galaxy, somewhere else, but if you have that instrument then you can catch the sound and hear it again. If you know someone recited the Namokar mantra at a certain time and place, you can focus that instrument there and you might be able to hear that sound millions of years later. You can catch the frequency. If we can catch sound in a voice recorder from two feet away, what's wrong with catching it two million miles away with a better instrument? It's just a matter of time. It takes time to go from someone's voice to a tape recorder, even if it's only half of a second. So, it doesn't matter if it's a million years later you can still catch the sound. Nothing is impossible.

You have to recite the divine sounds from the navel. It's a deep sound, and the deep sound comes from the depth of your body. It will create more electricity, more vibration and purity. Never recite through your throat like Tibetans do. It doesn't have much effect. It's not a natural sound and doesn't create the right vibrations. I don't know why Buddhists have a lot of illusion. They have a very good sound, but they speak it through their throats: *Om Mani Padme Hum.* "Mani" means "center," and they still don't get it. I don't blame them, because they don't have sounds that come from the navel more in their language, so they don't learn to recite the proper way. If the language doesn't have it, where will they learn it?

By reciting loudly it will create more electricity, so there is a bigger benefit. When you do it like that, your thoughts disappear quicker and the mind will cooperate. But when you recite by your mind only, you begin to think about things and your mind can go here and there. It requires more focus and experience. If you do the Namokar mantra out loud only five times, and recite a whole mala, 108 times, in your mind, the ones you did loudly might be even better than the whole mala. There is a time that you can't recite loudly though, like if there are people nearby and by reciting you might be disturbing them. Maybe they're sleeping or working, or some other thing. Then it's not right to do it. Do them in your mind if you might disturb people at that time. If nobody is near you, or if you are outside in nature, then you can do them loudly. When you're disturbing others, even if you're doing good things, then it's not right. Regardless of if you are doing the mantras in your mind or out loud, when you do mantras whole-heartedly, without expectation – that is the best.

MUDRAS

A *mudra* is like a yoga posture for your hands. Our nervous system connects through all parts of our bodies up to our brain. From our toes, through our feet, our hands, up to our brain. Our hands have more nerves so we can discern between different sensations and feelings, like hotness or warmth, if something is rough or smooth. Your hands will tell you a lot; they have very sensitive nerves and many blood vessels. Your feet won't tell you as much. If your thoughts are becoming hyper, going here and there with no calmness, the mudras will calm your mind down. The brain is affected by certain positions of the hand.

Mudras are very ancient, coming from the Samanic tradition, the monks and nuns. If someone has a lot of difficulty doing yoga postures, they can learn mudras with less difficulty and it will help them. I'm talking about if a person's body won't allow them to do that kind of stretching, because of course you will have difficulty in the beginning of practicing yoga if you have never stretched your body like that before. Mudras help the brain and mind by releasing toxins, similar to yoga postures. Sometimes when you have pains in your arms or hands then they can help with that, too.

They are important to practice, but young people who can gain flexibility should try to do yoga postures and mudras together, like sitting in lotus posture and creating a mudra at the same time will create even more energy. And if you recite a mantra on top of that, you won't believe how much energy you can make in your body.

You have to be careful with the position of your hands and fingers, the way you place them. If you have your palm open and facing away from you, but it's not touching any of your body like the edge of your knee, then the energy goes out. It has to touch your body, even if it's the backside of your hand. That's the way you keep energy locked in your system and it builds up.

When our fingers are placed in these different positions, they affect us because they become like yin and yang. The energy that is going to be wasted if your hands and fingers are open is sent back into you. Most of the time our hands are releasing energy because we're unaware of the system. When you do certain positions it all goes back into your body, like a circuit. The mudra is creating a circuit to keep your electricity in. Unless you're in the highest state of consciousness, then your hands will only suck energy in, and never release it. Even if you're holding a book in your hands that is considered closed, because the energy can go through the material back into your fingers.

Make sure you are closing your system only when you need the extra energy. When you're meditating, you better close it because the energy will flow in you and not be wasted. In meditation we need a lot of energy. When we touch the index and thumb together, it flows back in. Or, you can sit with your right hand over the left.

Our index finger is the most important. You have to know about it. The index finger, or pointer, is called the *tarjani*, the influential finger. It has a lot of influence. If someone points their finger at you and says something like, "Stop, don't do it!" They're influencing you, right? Why? Because this finger releases and sucks a lot of energy, much more than any of the other fingers. If negative people are around you, it will suck in that negative energy, so don't seek the company of any negative people. All fingers suck in energy, but the index does it very quickly. It can bring a lot of energy in, and also release it quickly, too. Remember this when you are using a mala to count your mantras. A mala is a 108-beaded rosary. You never want to touch the mala with your index finger – never do it. It will suck all the energy from the mala, just the opposite of what you want to do. You want the mala to be full of energy and create that kind of positive vibration in you when you are practicing with it.

Our hands create heat in certain positions – a lot of electricity. When you release a mudra, suddenly you feel the blood circulation flow better. That is the way to heal yourself. You have to sit in the mudra, not just for one minute, it doesn't work that way. Stay with the mudra for 20 minutes, or 30 minutes. That works.

Remember the vyana vayu, the prana which is everywhere throughout the body. It begins to flow inside the body rather than leaking out after you become experienced with mudras. Some are difficult and can take even six months to learn them perfectly. Vyana is like electricity; if you don't use it, it will go out. Mudras will keep it flowing in the body. You block it from leaving from your index finger and it flows back into you. We use a lot of prana this way that would otherwise be wasted.

Mudras are not so difficult, but you have to practice and put effort to feel the effects. It's even better if you combine them with postures or mantras and meditation. You can protect yourself with the mudras. You don't have to make it obvious; if you're around some negative people and it's affecting you, you close your system by just making a slight fist, or touch the fingers together, or touching your hand on the side of your leg. It is better to lock all the fingers by touching them together, but it will work by simply touching your body, too. This way maybe they won't notice you are even doing anything.

In Part III, I will share with you which specific mudras will activate and balance each of your chakras and in Part IV you can see the images.

PART III:
TECHNIQUES
OF THE CHAKRA SYSTEM

THE CHAKRAS

When I'm asked about the chakras, the most common question is, "Why did they give the name of chakra?" In Sanskrit, chakra simply means "wheel." The chakra is a wheel. The energy in our bodies moves like a wheel, clockwise, and in an area that is merely two inches in diameter. The energy doesn't move like in many pictures that people create, showing that our chakras are very wide; that is just radiance only. If the energy moves very slowly, it means your chakra is blocked and having some difficulties in being balanced. If the energy doesn't move too fast, or too slow, then it means this chakra is working properly. You don't want the energy to move too quickly, because the chakra becomes over-active and will give you just as much trouble as if it's blocked.

If you feel sick, or if you feel pain somewhere in your body, or your organs and glands are not functioning properly, you'll learn how to make them very healthy with the chakra system. Remember, this system originated from Parshvanath, the 23rd Tirthankara, 2,900 years ago, and will help you move closer to the spiritual path that can bring you to enlightenment, and finally liberation from all of your pains, sorrows, and suffering as you go up and down in your life. There is not one person who doesn't suffer; unless they are in the highest state of consciousness, everybody suffers in their own ways. On the surface it may look as if someone has a very extraordinary life – a lot of success, creativity, friends and so on – but that is just the appearance. It's like packaging, and when you open it up you find out there are many pieces that are broken and it's not what you expected to find inside the box. It's better to not pay attention to the packaging, and instead, find the meaning in your life. On this tiny planet in our galaxy, which is just one out of countless galaxies among the stars, why are you here? What's stopping you from finding out? That is all you have to do. Awaken your soul. All of your suffering will dissolve and the whole universe becomes crystal-clear to you. It is difficult, that is sure, but it's possible. When you can clean your system out and balance your chakras, you will begin to move towards that. You begin to see what your existence really is, and it's beautiful. In the Samanic tradition of monks and nuns, it is the purest tradition, because they're always seeking to improve themselves in order to dissolve their karma. They take responsibility for their mistakes in the past and remain balanced as they go through the suffering that comes back to them. They accept it and don't let it affect them. That is the way to be awakened. You'll find by yourself what you need to do because the energy is flowing upwards; a sudden change happens in you.

So, this energy moves like a wheel, but it has to move with enough current, enough force. If it doesn't move speedily enough, then the chakra will not be active and you'll see what it brings in your life. Your moods will be up and down, your thoughts will be unclear. When the energy is moving too quickly, then the chakra has too much energy and creates other symptoms that make a person very scattered and they can't stay still anytime.

The techniques I give are very safe, and they were taught by the monks and nuns thousands of years ago. The system has diminished, but people are becoming interested in it again after all this time. You need to understand all of these things when you begin practicing to awaken your chakras. It's a very easy-to-follow system, and when your chakras are balanced your life will transform. You will be very joyful, peaceful and balanced.

"Why does our energy flow downward?" This is the second question I'm asked about chakras and kundalini. Energy is like water, and the nature of water is to flow downward. If you want to make the water flow upward you have to do a lot of things; you might have to create a dam, or change the terrain for the water to flow a different way. Remember, it is not an easy thing to change the current of the water to flow upward. It takes a lot of effort. That's why the yogic system is a very difficult system to follow, unlike Parshvanath's system. In the yogic system they don't talk about your intention much, and how it affects you. Parshvanath used the leshyas to show people what their actions and intentions were like, and what can happen when they begin to think higher. If your energy flows downward your chakras will be very weak. There isn't enough speed in the energy for it to jump up to the next chakra. If the first chakra is weak, then how will the others have any energy? It begins with the root chakra, our base.

PARSHVANATH: THE LESHYAS

Parshvanath was teaching about the leshyas, intentions, and how to bring them higher and higher to become very pure. Our intentions can create a lot of trouble in our lives, because when they're combined with our words and actions we will get the result of those intentions. If our intentions are polluted by anger, jealousy, desires and other such qualities, then that is the way we will speak and act. When we understand why our intentions are not pure, we can work to improve them, and as a result of doing so, we raise the energy in our chakras at the same time.

The color red is for survival. Parshvanath was teaching that without the *Tejo leshya*, you cannot survive. This red is like the red of a sunrise, and it brings heat and pranic-force. Without pranic-force, you cannot survive. The Tejo leshya is connected to the first chakra and creates self-preservation, because it gives you the power to sustain yourself. It grounds you. If there is no fire in your body, no heat or activity, then your body won't be alive. Red can bring you tremendous energy and reduce your cravings to eat much food. When you have heat in your body, it gives you the feeling that you're here, in your body, and you have to survive and sustain yourself. This is where your physical identity is created. Without much pranic-force, when you have a very low Tejo leshya, you'll feel a lot of fear, heaviness, and laziness. You'll have a slow metabolism and feel a lot of greediness. It's what happens when the first chakra is not active enough, when there is not much force moving in it. When a person feels fear, is undisciplined, underweight, or feeling disconnected and spacey, these are all symptoms that the kundalini is very low in the first chakra, and it shows they have a low Tejo leshya. How can you increase your leshya here? Tejo leshya is the fifth leshya; the person is shaking the branches of the mango tree and has a higher intention, but not yet the highest. If you increase this intention in you, it will activate the first chakra more and more. Eat early in the evening, go to sleep early, wake up early and watch the sunrise. The red of the sunrise will help you. "Namo Siddhanam," will create tremendous light and color so that the first chakra is activated properly.

The leshya connected with both the second and third chakra is the *Padma leshya*. Its color is pink, yellowish and orange. If you don't have enough orange color in your body, the second chakra will create a lot of sexual desires, self-gratifying actions and many emotions. Orange light is created when you recite, "Namo Aayariyaanaṁ." This will help the kundalini flow better in your second chakra. This chakra holds the feeling that you want someone, because it's considered the emotional center, or emotional identity. You can feel a lot of guilt when there is not much energy here, and become very attached to someone, easily addicted into sexual behavior or other experiences that bring you enjoyment. A person can also become emotionally numb and fearful of pleasure if the energy is going the wrong way. Desires are not balanced or healthy when the energy is slow in this chakra. To increase energy in this chakra and balance your emotions then you have to work on increasing your Padma leshya.

The third chakra creates the color yellow which is a very powerful color. Yellow creates a strong will and self-definition of who you really are. Spontaneity, self-esteem and vitality all increase when a person has a lot of yellow in them. These things come when your intention is more pure and the second chakra is balanced. The Padma leshya makes you act. If your intention is not yet increased to Padma leshya and your second chakra is weak, then it is very difficult for you to take action with your decisions. When yellow is lacking, the person will begin to identify with their ego and also have feelings of shame. They become very scattered, have an aggressive or dominating nature, or become weak-willed and fearful. Padma leshya needs to be increased and the third chakra needs to have more yellow light. Reciting, "Namo Aayariyaanaṁ," will also help create yellow energy.

Neel leshya has the dark blue and dark green colors. It relates to the fourth chakra. When there is enough dark green in your body this chakra will be very healthy and you will have tremendous love and very healthy relationships. The quality of self-acceptance is created in you. A person can become a social butterfly, because the heart chakra creates the social identity. When green is lacking in a person, they become jealous and very possessive, shy, lonely, bitter and isolated. Think about it, and work on increasing your Neel leshya.

The fifth chakra is the throat chakra, and it's related to the *Krishan leshya*. Krishan leshya has a grey-blue color, like a pigeon. When you have enough of this color, you're able to communicate very well with other people. You have self-expression, clear communication and creativity. Creativity belongs to this chakra. When your intention is not raised up to the Krishan leshya yet, then you'll find it hard to be creative. When you recite, "Namo Loe Savva Sahunaṁ," it automatically begins to activate the fifth chakra. What's going to happen if there is not enough of this grey-blue color in someone? The person will lie often and keep themselves in illusion. Even if they want to tell the truth, they'll tell the lie; when the color is lacking they can't say the truth. That person will be talking non-stop and have little or no listening skills when they're with other people. When they speak, the words won't sound good together and they'll make confusing statements or keep changing what their story is while they're telling it. They have a poor rhythm when speaking.

Another leshya related to the fifth chakra is *Kapota leshya*, because the color is similar. In the Jain system it's described as tasting an unripe mango; it's very stringent and difficult to digest. If this chakra is not active enough it will create those kind of unripe feelings in a person. Their color becomes heavy, because their intention is that way. When a person's intention is in Kapota leshya, it means the fifth chakra is not active. You have to bring your intention out of Kapota leshya, into the Padma leshya. You transform slowly, that's the way you grow higher and higher. Awaken this chakra slowly.

The sixth chakra has the color of indigo, dark blue, so, it's related to the *Neel leshya* also. When this chakra is active, you have a lot of intuition, imagination and the quality of self-reflecting. When the chakra is really open, it creates true psychic perception. By reciting, "Namo Uvajjhayaanaṁ," it creates a lot of indigo color and balances this chakra. You begin to see the truth and understand things clearly. When a person lacks indigo in their body, it creates a false identity for them. They won't recognize who they are. The most visible symptoms are: nightmares, headaches, hallucinations, no concentration, difficult memories and unwillingness to accept things.

The seventh chakra is related to the *Shukal leshya*. If you have enough white light in your body it creates a lot of awareness in you. Shukal leshya is the best intention that you can have; you don't want to harm anything or anyone. When your Sahasrara chakra is active, you gain self-knowledge, which is never-ending. It brings wisdom, spiritual visions and communication. You begin to know yourself, who you really are. To increase white in this chakra, recite, "Namo Arihantaanaṁ." The way it's written creates white light. Once there is white light in you, the seventh chakra activates by itself and you get out of your box; you get the universal identity. If you're following any religion, you'll leave that box. If you're Catholic, Christian, Jain, Hindu, Muslim, Buddhist, you'll leave that box. You begin to open up when you have the universal identity. When this chakra is blocked, when you're not in the Shukal leshya, it creates a lot of attachment, and will take the person from life to life, continuously wandering. Sometimes when the energy here is too much, the person can become over-intellectual. They begin to think that other people don't know anything, that they're the only one who knows. Spiritual addiction is not good either. It's like confusion. Be careful and make sure this chakra is always active. If it's blocked somehow, you'll have learning difficulties, remain always skeptical, have rigid thinking and be materialistic. These things will take over you.

You have to go little by little, through each leshya. Combine the leshyas with the chakra system and you'll be surprised how quickly they begin to open. Remember that leshya is your intention, and it needs to be purified. Bring your leshya to the Shukal leshya and you'll be in bliss and ecstasy. Then you'll be a real devotee of Parshvanath. Otherwise, you just sing the song in his praise, but you don't even follow the system he taught. Remember the symbol of the first kundalini master, the seven-hooded snake, reminding you to raise your kundalini energy, raise your intention and become the purest; become a liberated soul.

The origin of the Ganges River is known as *Gangotri*. It flows down from the Himalayas and towards the ocean. To lift your energy back up through your chakras is comparable to the water in the ocean going all the way back up the Ganges to Gangotri in the Himalayas – some of the highest peaks on the earth. That's what Parshvanath was teaching. Transform your anger. Transform your greed and negativities, your jealousy and ego. These are the symptoms you need to take care of. Otherwise your dhara, the current that naturally flows down, will never turn into radha, the path. Or, there is another way: you can evaporate the water and make a cloud of it, and it will float even higher than the Himalayas where it originated. But without efforts you cannot do anything. That's why your energy flows down, because you're stuck in your lower qualities.

BEGINNING YOUR PRACTICE

I will tell you that it's not safe to work on your chakras if you are trying by yourself. When you are practicing under the guidance of a true enlightened master, someone who has reached the highest state of consciousness, then it is safe. The real master will know the meaning of the teachings and have insight into the techniques and how they affect you. They can see what is happening in you. It must be a real master, not simply a person you believe to be a master. Maybe they aren't the real thing. Under the guidance of a master it is safe to activate your chakras.

I will mention everything that is necessary, but before you begin to activate your chakras you need to know where the energy is moving, and I will go one by one. Remember, there is a big misconception of chakras. Physically speaking, they don't exist; it is just the area where energy is moving in you. The chakra is referring to that area. This energy is very powerful; it can show you a lot of spiritual visions, and make you an extraordinary person. If you're not a strong person, you can become very strong. If you're not an intelligent person, you can become very intelligent.

When you are finished going through this book and understanding it deeply, you will feel that nothing is impossible in this world. You have the ability to do it. You have the strength to do it, the courage to do it and the power to do it. You need to awaken it. Nothing is impossible; this word is wrong. You need to see it as "I'm possible." If a yogi can awaken their chakras, what is wrong with you? Why can't you do it? You need to just find the person who has the experience and knowing to give you the right guidance and techniques.

If someone is just beginning to learn and understand about the chakra system and how the energy is working in their body, I suggest a very important first step. Before you can really achieve the growth you're looking for, you need to focus on food. What foods are you eating? I've mentioned several times that the human body is a super-instrument, and the only body you can achieve liberation with. It has to be very healthy. Free of pollution. So, the first thing you have to do is focus on changing the way you are giving energy to this instrument. It needs light food, we call it *sattvic* food. Sattvic food means divine food; it nourishes the body and creates the real temple which Parshvanath was teaching about. When you eat only the lightest foods, your body becomes pure, you never will feel any heaviness, laziness or lethargy, and your thoughts become very positive automatically. Otherwise if you're eating foods that don't give all the best nutrients then how can you expect to see results from your chakra practices? It's all related. It is a system and it has to be followed carefully. It is very simple when you become familiar with it, and you will see your life transform. If you can be aware of all the things you eat and drink, you are taking a big step.

Don't eat any meats; it creates so much heaviness and brings many toxins into the body. Any kind of smoking, drinking alcohol, using drugs or too many medicines will do a lot of damage to your body. There is no way you can successfully raise your energy while you're under the influence of any substance, or if your body is full of those toxins. It's not possible. Think about it; if heavy foods can bring your energy down, what do you think those substances will do to you? They can even do permanent damage to your nadis that is irreversible. No sadhana or yoga practice can take back that kind of damage you've done to your own body. It is very important you take care of your instrument.

The second step is to then work on positive thinking. This is the best way. You transform your thoughts from negative and heavy thoughts, to lighter and more positive thoughts. What do you want to achieve in your life? You can do it. You need to have a positive attitude if you want to take yourself higher and higher. If you're always flowing in negative thoughts, worries and feeling nervous and anxious, your energy is flowing down and down. If you can change your foods from heavy to light and have positive thoughts, that will begin to change your life right away and your chakras will start to open by themselves. Anything positive helps raise your kundalini energy.

Chakras are important on the spiritual path, but it is not necessarily going to take you to your goal. Your goal is supposed to be liberation. Someone cannot merely work on their chakras and reach enlightenment. Even if a person is working very seriously, it will only make them very healthy and very light in the body. They will feel like they are floating and have very pure thoughts, but that is just the beginning. Then they can work on the real sadhana and dive deep into their consciousness to see what they really are. If all the chakras are balanced it helps you to feel very joyful, content, have good health and you can gain a lot of understanding (if you have the right guidance), because your mind is clear. Your body will begin to cooperate with you and you can go further towards enlightenment. Don't be confused that you can get enlightened by working on your chakras and kundalini only. That is a wrong idea, and whoever is teaching that is misleading you.

When you begin practicing these techniques to awaken your chakras and raise your energy, it takes a minimum of 21 days for you to see any result, but 41 days is normal. You have to do consistent practice. This is how long it takes to move one or two layers of toxins in your body, shake them fully and burn them. If you are only doing your practice every few days then it will take longer to see what kind of effect it has on you, so make sure you are putting the effort and doing the work. Don't be lazy. It is one thing to be on the spiritual path, but to move forward on the path is a difficult task; it takes a lot of patience and courage. I always tell people that God helps those who help themselves, and it's true. What will happen if you just sit around waiting for something to happen to you? It doesn't work like that. So put the effort to awaken your chakras and you will see what can happen. All the toxins are blocking the way for your kundalini to flow and they need to be forced out. The less clean your body is, the lesser chance you have to open the chakras.

If the lower three chakras are blocked, then you need to start by working on them first. The energy isn't available somehow, and you have to create it before it can begin to flow upward. Don't jump to the higher chakras right away, because if the energy is not there in the bottom three, how will it go up in the first place?

You will see all the symptoms of the chakras being balanced, blocked, or over-active, and you can compare them to see how yours are doing. If you don't think that you have these symptoms in you, then it's an indication that maybe the chakra is not blocked and you can work on the next one. If you're really working hard and after 41 days you begin to feel a big change and you feel some kind of balance then compare the symptoms and see if you need to work on the chakra more, or if you can move on. When the chakras are all 80% active and balanced, the person is supposed to feel joyful and even if they eat or if they don't eat, the person is not bothered at all. They feel peaceful and balanced. The body needs food to survive, but the person's mind will not be disturbed if they have to go without eating for some time. If a chakra is blocked you have to work hard, and sometimes the energy can be moving the wrong way in the body. When energy is not moving the right way a person will feel crazy, maybe scream often, have too much anger, big headaches and different pains throughout the body. It means the energy is not going upward, and it may be going somewhere else in the body. You have to stop your practice right away and seek the guidance of a real master.

CHAKRA BLOCKAGES

A blockage means the energy doesn't move in that area, or if it's moving then it's very slow. If the movement is very slow, the energy can't jump up to the next chakra because there's no force. It's like trying to jump ten feet off the ground but you only have enough energy to get up on the tips of your toes. When energy moves very slow, you feel you are in your body and you might be busy doing a lot of things but you don't enjoy anything, everything feels heavy to you.

It's not good to have a blocked chakra and it can cause a lot of complications in your life because it affects your health as well as your thoughts and communication. Energy cannot stop moving completely, because the person will be dead then. It only moves slowly. When someone's energy stops moving altogether, then they will die. Nobody's chakras are 100% blocked, maybe only 70%. Energy is there, but it's not healthy. Your main nadis will not be clear when your chakras are blocked. You will never flow in balance, always staying in emotions or anger, frustration and over-excitement and restlessness.

Your brain is squeezed between two chakras, the 6th and 7th chakras. So, the brain will not communicate with you what is right and what is wrong. You'll spend all day and night in your attachments and it will keep you from doing any spiritual practices. That's why when your chakras are really blocked, your mind is not clear so you can't be aware that anything is even wrong in you. To love someone is different from attachment, but you won't be able to see the difference. Blockages can be caused by your lower emotions; getting trapped in them too much and not understanding them. Or, by indulging in sex too much. Heavy foods, negative thinking, always watching negative things on the T.V. or in movies. All these things make your energy flow downward and it makes your chakras remain asleep. It's better to be on the path and not put in your body things that stay in your system too long and damage your body. When you seriously work to clear the chakras, the blockages will begin to dissolve. It won't bring difficult experiences like emotional turmoil, unless that is a result of the new change you go through. It is all temporary. The symptoms begin to clear away and you feel lighter and fresh like you just woke up from a long sleep. If you are angry a lot, then you'll feel the opposite once the blockage begins to dissolve.

Diseases are a combination of karma and chakras being imbalanced. Sometimes the chakras are blocked because of your habits and not necessarily your karma. You have a lot of habits. It can be over-eating, even if you're eating good food you can still eat too much, or too much sugar, too much caffeine. Even if you're a vegetarian and stay away from drinking and other things, you still have to be careful and watch your habits. Mostly it is habits that block your chakras. Sometimes the karma creates it and you have that kind of weak body that feels heavy. Habits don't necessarily come from karma; you can create new ones by your current thoughts and attitudes. Like a baby watches their parents and surroundings and learns that way, they create a lot of habits from that. If someone in your family is helping poor people, maybe you'll develop that

good habit just by watching them. If someone is hunting, or comes home from work and drinks beer all night, you will build a bad habit by watching them. The society, instead of helping us, gives us the wrong ideas most of the time. People get trapped into it and that's how you can create the habits that take you the wrong way. If society begins to understand a lot of things, the family is supposed to be very healthy and happy and they will develop only new good habits. It's the human's nature to indulge into bad things quickly, but with good things it takes them time. Sometimes a blockage cannot be removed because your karma has given you that kind of body. Maybe it's always sick or too weak, so you cannot get rid of the blockage. That, you can blame on your karma. Your karma is simply giving you the result of what you did in the past. If you keep working on your health and find ways of alternative medicines, natural medicines, it will help your body to be in better health even with those sicknesses, and your chakras will have a better chance of opening because of the lack of chemicals.

The best way to break blockages in the chakras is by reciting the sounds that I give in this book. Then the yoga postures and the water technique. These are very strong and will help the most. If your practice is consistent you can expect a lot of good results. A lot of times people can have blocked chakras because of the culture and society they live in. If a person is raised on meat in their culture, then their chakras will be very blocked, all the way down to the first chakra. Native Americans for example, they are mostly living on reservations, but what do they do there? They drink and smoke even more. Few people get out of there and they begin to see how society works and they might begin to work hard. They stop drinking and smoking tobacco. Even good people, the native people, are damaging their bodies by doing that all the time. This is how cultures can create blockages in the chakras. It can be the opposite way, too: people can have more balanced chakras from their culture. It has to be more of a farming culture. Where there are people farming and working a lot, their first chakras will work better because they're with nature most of the time and being very active. Suppose Texas, even though they consume a lot of meat, there are a lot of farmers here, so their first chakras will be more balanced than people in big cities. But because of eating meat, their other chakras will have problems. In India, if you go there, they go to the temple in the morning and listen to the *satsang*, the spiritual teachings, and it gives them good thoughts throughout the day. That is their daily routine, so by the time they become negative, it's time to go to the temple and start the next day. It can help them be more balanced by hearing good things and being in positive thinking. A tribal person is supposed to have more balanced chakras, but if they're violent or harming their body by smoking marijuana, drinking or using drugs, then it will be the opposite. No matter if they live 24 hours a day in nature, their chakras will be fully blocked. In the very old period of time, tribal living was eating more fruits and roasting vegetables, and even though they were hunting, they were roaming in the forests all day long so they got a lot of exercise and their bodies were strong. Tribal living is good when they don't fight so much and kill each other. Nowadays, people who live on farms and grow their own foods are even better than tribal living. Maybe a medicine man in the native tribe is in better shape, because they're trying to heal other people so their thoughts are more positive. In Africa, tribal living is not the same way. They have a lot of violence in many tribes and carry rituals that are torturous. When the young boys have to get a circumcision it is torture and cruel to them. They don't have any relief from it – no numbness at all. They think it is to become a man, to be brave. It's torture, and they have many chances to get sick and become infected by doing this. In that kind of experience your first chakra can become very shocked and it can create a big blockage that will be hard to clear. Many tribal things are not good. When you're working on your chakras, go through them one at a time and try to feel what is happening. You will see the results.

MULADHARA: THE FIRST CHAKRA

If the energy in the first chakra doesn't move then you won't be active in life. It is called *Muladhara*. In Sanskrit, it means the "root," the "base." It's the root chakra; people often refer to it as this. If this chakra is somehow blocked, you don't have the basic energy to get up and do something. How will you raise your kundalini to your crown chakra if there is no force in the Muladhara? This is where you create the dam, and it builds and builds until there's enough force to go upward.

You need tremendous energy in the root, an incredible amount of energy. The Muladhara chakra is located at the base of the spine, and I mentioned that the chakras are just two inches in diameter. This is where the energy is moving. From a medical point of view, there are two glands you can check, and if they're healthy it means the energy here is moving at the right speed and in the right direction. No matter how much food or protein you put in your body, you will feel drained and heavy if the energy in the Muladhara is unhealthy. You have to check the suprarenal and adrenal glands on the kidneys. They sit there, like a cap; on the left side of the kidney is the suprarenal gland, and on the right is the adrenal gland. If they're not working properly, they won't hold any energy. When the chakra has no energy, the bladder can be very sick, or the kidneys and the spine can be hurt. This means the energy is not moving. Here are the symptoms of the energy in this area. You can use them to see how healthy your Muladhara chakra is.

Active Symptoms:

Grounded. Do you feel grounded in your life?

Stable. Do you have stability in your life?

Security. Financial security, security with friends and family; they are indications of what kind of life your energy is creating.

No distrust. You don't have problems trusting, or hold distrust against anyone.

Present moment. Do you live in the past, the future, or are you able to live in the present?

Connected with physical body. Do you treat your body well? Do you care about it and feel like it is part of you?

Inactive Symptoms:

Fearful. You are always living in your fears.

Nervousness. You feel nervous very often.

Unwelcoming to others. You are not gracious with people.

Negativity. Your mind is mostly taken by negative thoughts.

Jealousy. Do you find yourself feeling jealous often?

Anger. You feel frustration and anger.

Sexual desires. Either physically or in your thoughts, you indulge in sexual desires too much.

Overactive Symptoms:

Materialistic. You constantly think of your belongings and getting new things, even if you don't really need them.

Greediness. You want more things for yourself, and think of yourself before considering other people.

If you follow the system I am sharing with you, you can balance your Muladhara chakra. The element of the first chakra is the earth. Live near the earth; live with nature, live in a clean area. If you live away from lots of pollution the Muladhara will open automatically, but if you live in a concrete jungle, it will be blocked more easily. There is no earth in the concrete jungle. It can be rivers, or the ocean, forests, mountains or deserts; it's all nature. Earth will stimulate the Muladhara chakra. If you can find large red rocks, maybe in the western United States for example, if you stay on them while practicing meditation it will create a lot of energy. Or, you can simply sit on a red blanket, or red dirt. If you can find a forest with a lot of pine trees, they will create that kind of red energy in you even if you meditate below them for just thirty minutes. Most people who come here to Siddhayatan have a blocked first chakra. It's because many people live in the concrete jungle. They are not with nature. In the big cities, they have a problem with this, and they keep locking themselves in. The Muladhara chakra needs nature and earth to remain balanced. If those people never take time to be with nature then they will be in trouble. Go to the lake, go to the forest, go somewhere where there is no pollution, or less pollution. In Manhattan and New York City, there are some areas but it's mostly clouded with too much pollution. But people also don't have much time to spend either. It's better to live a simple life and not live in big, multi-story buildings made of concrete and steel. It blocks your first chakra. It's not enough just to see nature from your window; you have to be there. Earth is vital for creating energy in the Muladhara, so make sure that you put effort to be with nature if you don't happen to live there already. If you're serious about working on your chakras then you will make the time for it. You will begin to feel very grateful for life and become a down-to-earth person, because you are already bringing yourself to be with the earth.

This energy can also be created by sound, and there are two sounds which create the vibration the root chakra needs. The first sound is "*lam*." It's not pronounced like the English word "lamb." In Sanskrit there are thirteen vowels, and in English there are only five. One of the Sanskrit vowels is "ṁ." It makes a nasal sound, like the ending of the word "lung." That's how you make the sound of this vowel. When you can pronounce this sound the right way, it sounds similar to the word "lung." You will see this sound again with the other chakras. If you recite this sound for just two to three minutes, it will create a lot of heat at the base of the spine and begin to create energy and movement in the Muladhara chakra. This is a well-known sound but very few people know how to pronounce it the right way.

The second sound is a very powerful and divine sound. You won't be able to find it anywhere else for the chakras because nobody knows these sounds. The sound is "*daakini.*" "Daa" is the sound, and "kini" is the cap. When you say, "daa," the first chakra opens up and the energy gains speed. It will keep going so you need to put the cap on it. "Kini" is the cap to close the sound and keep the energy there. You have to pronounce it the right way; it's very long. It's not like you just read it here and repeat it as a little word. When you say, "daa," it has to be very long, like this: daaaaaaaaaaaaaaaaaa. You take a deep breath to start with, and when you're ready you recite it very powerfully: daaaaaaaaaaaaaaaaaakini. It might take you five to ten seconds to recite this sound. The closing cap, "kini," sounds the same as "key," and "knee." If you have any symptoms that the Muladhara is blocked, then recite this sound all the time, at least 108 times each day, and it will really clear out any blockages. If you would like to hear and learn the correct pronunciation for this chakra (and all chakras) visit http://chakraawakeningbook.com/suite.

Every chakra is ruled by some power of God. The power of the Muladhara is creative power. In Hindu culture, creative power is called Brahma. If you make an effort to concentrate on creativity, the chakra will balance and open more. You can be creative in the kitchen, on the computer, in writing, music and art, business, sports; you can be creative anywhere. Creativity is very important in our lives. You have to understand, who has power is not the same as the power itself. They are separate. If you are holding a glass of water, it might be your water, but it's separate from you. Somebody can have a lot of intelligence and society might call them a genius or a scientist. The intelligence, or maybe writing, is their power, and they are separate. In the same way, God is creative, but it is not God, it's only an aspect of God. We call it Brahma – it's symbolic. Put all of your energy in creativity. If you're always in creation, doing new things and putting effort into that, then you will have a lot of energy in life. Even if you're simply reading; put your own understanding there and it becomes like your new way of ideas, a new concept. Even thinking can be creative. Sometimes the Hindus think their stories are literal, but they are merely symbolic. They show all the Gopis dancing around Krishna while he plays the flute. Hindus are mesmerized by his flute and they forgot the real meaning of it. Krishna was a very joyful person when he was alive, and they wanted to find a way to show that kind of joy in the pictures, so they made all the images of the girls dancing around him while he plays music. It was just a way to show his happiness, but look what the Hindus are doing. It means be happy and joyful like Krishna. There was no way to show that kind of happiness in a picture, so they made it this way and Hindus take it literally. That's the way things get distorted and the meaning is not understood any longer. So, the power of God is separate from God. When we visualize this creativity and indulge in it, we can transform ourselves. It can be just thinking, reading, or visualizations even. It's all creation.

All of these techniques and concepts will help activate the Muladhara chakra if you go deep into them. The sense of the first chakra is the sense of smell. You remember in really hot weather when a strong rain comes, it's pouring down heavily, and after the clouds have passed by there is a beautiful smell released in the air; the smell of the wet earth. This is the best smell to help balance the Muladhara. The first chakra is a grounding force and belongs more to physical matter, so the earth helps the chakra to become very strong. That is the best kind of smell for this chakra, full of the fragrance of the earth.

Herbs and spices can be used to help the chakras, too. You can cook with them in your meals and combine them with other fruits and vegetables that will help the chakra as well. Or you can simply use them for fragrance, which will help this chakra, as it's sense is smell. When you have raw turmeric you can mix it in a soup, or eat it with vegetables – that will help a lot. It grows underground and when you take it out it looks like ginger. Red chilies help because of the heat, or green chilies if they're very hot. But don't eat them with every meal, or even every day. Twice a week will do enough help. You don't want to overdo it when eating very spicy foods, because it can damage your body. There is a flower called *palash pushpa*, and it blossoms on the hottest days of the year. In India, it's usually May and June. If you find some of these flowers when they're dry, put them into a piece of cloth and you can place the cloth on top of the place where you meditate. When you're doing your meditation practice it will help create that grounding energy.

If you have a garnet crystal, blood ruby or a blood stone, these all have elements which help open your chakra. Wear them on a necklace, or as small pieces in rings if you don't want to wear a necklace. You can put the stones on the base of your spine, just touch it there for a few moments, or even sleep with the stones there. It gives energy and warmth to stimulate the kundalini there. Metals also help: copper, iron, titanium, zinc and aluminum.

Yoga postures, asanas, create a lot of energy that the body needs to clear out the toxins and blockages that prevent the chakras from opening up. Kundalini will rise higher and higher, because the body is strong, and with the right diet, clean as well. Siddhasana is the best posture for the Muladhara. It's very difficult, but it's the way to awaken kundalini if you can master it. Many people don't know about Goduhasana – the cow – milking posture. Even just a couple of minutes in this posture creates a lot of energy in the root chakra. If the chakra is full of energy – high current, high force – it will push up to the second, third, fourth and so on. It has to be completely retained energy in order to push up. If the glands don't hold energy and work properly, it's hard to build up energy. When the energy is retained in these glands you'll feel very healthy. Bhunamanasana is a very important posture. It's considered both a mudra and a yoga posture. Padmasana, lotus posture, also helps but make sure that your spine remains erect in this position. Simhasana, the lion posture, creates so much energy if you can stay there. I mentioned to do it for 30 minutes; that is the mastery you need. Vrkshasana, the tree posture. It will help you to gain concentration, mental clarity and become a very grounded person, like a very strong tree. The mudra you can practice is *Bhu mudra;* close your pinky and ring fingers to touch with the tip of your thumb, and extend your index and middle finger straight out. It looks like the popular "peace-sign," except the thumb is touching to those two fingers.

Aromatherapy can work if you have the right things. You need sandalwood oil, or cedar wood oil. These really activate this chakra if you can use them often where you live. They hold the earthy fragrance which stimulate the Muladhara.

If you're disconnected and live in worldly thinking, then it's hard to relax your senses and mind to go within yourself. You can put in a pair of earplugs or noise-canceling headphones to help quiet down and not be distracted. This will help you be in a better place to hear the inner-sounds of the chakras. Or, you can try the natural way by closing your ears with your thumbs, and placing the rest of your fingers over your eyes or on your forehead. Either is okay.

The sounds of the chakras are very beautiful. They can be heard deep inside of you, and it gives you a sign that your chakras are beginning to open up and get a lot of energy.

Sit down after doing the Surya Bhedi pranayama for three to five minutes and close your eyes. Try to relax completely and focus only on what's inside. Don't hear the things around you, the things going on in the outside world. The sound you will hear for the first chakra is like a bumble-bee – a low, humming sound that sounds very deep. It is like a buzzing sound. This is the sound of the first chakra awakening, or in the process of awakening.

For this chakra to be active and incredibly strong, it's important to follow the next thing I will mention. Don't eat any meats. This includes fish and eggs. Meat means anything that comes from another's flesh. People think without meat they cannot get protein, but they are fully wrong. They have the totally wrong concept about it. A lot of protein is in these foods I will mention here for your first chakra, and it is the best kind of protein for your body. It will give only sattvic energy, and sattvic is the lightest energy. It means "divine." It won't make you feel any heaviness at all. Beets, yams, cherries, cabbage, watermelon, tomato, strawberries: any red or red-skinned fruits and vegetables. These will be very good for the Muladhara. Also, radish, red peppers, red onion, eggplant, red grapes, cranberries, raspberries rhubarb.

If you don't have many red blood cells in your blood then this kind of food will help you create that energy. Energy needs to flow. It has to move fast to flow up and sattvic foods, very light foods, will help you. Light food means that it's digested very quickly in your system and with ease. It's not like greasy foods, or fried foods that sit in your intestines for such a long time having trouble being digested. Another thing to activate this chakra is roots. All the roots are in the ground and receive so much energy from the earth. They absorb a lot of energy. If you happen to find these kind of edible roots, they have a lot of energy. Once in a while if you have it in your meal you'll get a boost of energy. There is also an herb called *malathi*, the liquorice root, and it creates the red color in you. Put just a little bit in one gallon of water and heat it. Add some salt and take an enema; this will clear a lot of blockages from your Muladhara chakra. The best fruit to eat is pomegranate. Not the one you buy at the grocery store, but a very fresh one. Make fresh juice from it and it will help you a lot. In that area where Parshvanath was teaching there were pomegranates everywhere.

Red is the color of Muladhara's energy. Red is a warm color and it creates a lot of heat in you and makes you very active. There are many ways to visualize this color coming to you. One way is to place your right hand on your forehead, and your left near the base of your spine. Close your eyes and see all the red light coming and entering into your hands, going into your body. You can do it without placing your hands, too, it is just another way to do it. Or, you can simply visualize red light in the base of your spine and after some time it will create heat there. The energy will move. You need to know the significance of the red color. Red is the element of fire, and without fire, everything is paralyzed. Nothing moves. It means that without heat there is no motion or activity in the body. Red stimulates and excites the nerves and bloodstream, and if there's a deficiency in your senses anywhere, if the prana is lacking somewhere, red will strengthen the senses and help them gain power. It's a very important color. Red activates the blood circulation, and can energize your liver. You can wear any red clothing, or at night sleep by a red light. If you sleep in red light you'll be surprised; your vascular system will become so strong, it will send the right messages to your brain. If you visualize that you are breathing in red light through your breath, and it's reaching all through your body, every part, it will reduce the heat in your body. Red is heat, but it reduces heat in your body. When you breathe in a color, it goes everywhere in your body, because the Swashoswash balprana is the breath and flows everywhere. When we visualize that it's carrying color with it, the breath will take the color with it and can heal many things. Visualization becomes actualization. First you imagine, then you visualize, then it becomes actual. If you have congestion it will clear the congestion and mucus. It can do many things, because it is the color of health. Many diseases can be healed if you know how to visualize the red color. Remember you have to practice the techniques I mentioned already to become strong in visualization, then it will become actualization.

Practice tratka first, to gain concentration power, and then use the candle lit in a dark room to become an expert in visualization. Some diseases and problems in the body that have the potential to be healed are anemia, bronchitis, some cases of paralysis, pneumonia, and constipation. If you have an inflammatory condition I don't recommend to use the red color. Also if you have emotional disturbances, I don't recommend it. It can take you the opposite way. If none of these things are bothering you then you are safe to use the color.

Another way is to visualize a deep-red colored lotus flower that has four petals. On each petal is written, aṁ, vaṁ, saṁ and shaṁ. In the center of the flower is a yellow square, with a golden upside-down triangle inside of it. In the triangle is written laṁ. The lotus is very heavy and big, it has to be carried on the back of an elephant. If you visualize this whole image it will activate your Muladhara.

If you find a glass bottle, a red glass bottle, clean it out completely so you can drink from it. Fill it with water and on a sunny day, place it in open sunlight early in the morning. Keep it there until the sun sets, and don't let it go into the shade. It needs to absorb a lot of the sun's light to work well. It has to be a deep red color of glass, not plastic. It doesn't work if the glass is not originally red, so don't try to paint it; it has a different effect. Throughout the day the sun will enter through the bottle into the water and it becomes solarized water. It becomes medicine. In the evening as the sun sets, bring it inside and drink it. You don't have to drink it right at that moment, but don't put it in the refrigerator or leave it overnight because it will lose the energy. Diseases might begin to heal by drinking this solarized water, and your energy will move the right way. It is a very powerful technique. The Muladhara will start to move very fast.

Parshvanath was teaching a lot of secrets about the chakras – 2,900 years ago it happened. Mostly they're lost now. If you see his statue with the seven-hooded cobra over his head, remember he was giving the system of how to awaken your kundalini. Sometimes you can find his statue in the standing position. This position is a secret of the Muladhara chakra. If your backbone is a little bit bent, it will take longer to open the chakra. It's called kayotsarga. Kayotsarga means "to leave behind." It's referring to the body. You have to leave the body behind, forget it completely. Not like you don't care about your body, but you go so deep into consciousness that you don't remember your body is even there.

For kayotsarga, you have to stand straight with the inner-edges of your feet touching against each other, your arms are straight against your side with your palms and fingers resting against your thighs, and your back is fully erect. Your shoulders are broad and the chest is open. You don't close your fists, and you don't look down or up, you look straight forward and remain alert. The Muladhara chakra will remain straight; no matter how you sit, even in lotus posture, it can still bend sometimes. Kayotsarga is the best position for activating the first chakra. Your body becomes like a pillar. It's special because it's also considered a mudra because of the hand and feet positions. When you're in this position, pull all of the reproductive and rectum muscles upward. Do it at least 108 times, and with each pull, recite "Namo Siddhaanaṁ." It will create a lot of energy and red light. It means you forget your body while you're standing, and you go deep and you see all the lights in your body, and go deeper and even see what else is there.

Always keep this chakra active, it's very important in your life. You can't expect the energy to go higher and higher if there is no energy to begin with. The Muladhara has the basic energy for life, and in that sense it gives you the physical identity, the feeling that you are alive in this body. The chakra needs to be so strong. The energy has to be pulled up against the current, from the ocean to the mountains. When you stand in kayotsarga, pull up the muscles in the rectum. When you become older, the muscles here relax and sometimes the bladder is not in good health, so you'll have to go to the bathroom all the time. If you pull up the muscles 108 times while standing in kayotsarga, your body will become stronger and stronger every day.

Mahavira, the 24th Tirthankara, had ego about following Parshvanath's teachings. Even though he was a Tirthankara, he couldn't reach enlightenment; it was always around him but he couldn't get it. Somehow his first chakra was blocked, and when he finally dissolved his ego he reached enlightenment. He knew already how to break his ego, but he had to do it still. On the day he reached enlightenment, he was sitting in cow-milking posture. He stayed in that position for three days and it finally happened. In the Jain religion they don't accept the idea of yoga, because they think that you're making your body beautiful and becoming attached to it. The healthy body is beautiful, and the healthy body is the real vehicle to awaken the chakras and be on the path. The real Jain system is a different thing from the Jain religion people know about. They got fully trapped into traditions and don't go anywhere with it. If you don't keep your body healthy, clean and active, then how do you expect to shine? Many traditional Jain monks and nuns look like they're coming from the age of cavemen because they never even wash their faces. They seem to be depressed, because they don't even follow the system taught by the

Tirthankaras who they make statues of. Practice these postures, cow-milking posture and kayotsarga, and you'll be surprised how quickly your first chakra awakens.

SVADHISTHANA: THE SECOND CHAKRA

Two inches above the first chakra is the second chakra, the *Svadhisthana* chakra, and its color is orange. "Sva" means "your own," and "adhisthana" is the "abode." Your own abode. It means it is your home. If this chakra doesn't function correctly, you'll experience a feeling of homelessness, even if you have a house and a job. It's a restless feeling, an imbalanced feeling. You have everything, but you feel like you have nothing. This is an important chakra because it has something to do with the emotions, how you can express yourself and the fear you feel. The second chakra is also called the sacral center sometimes, because it is the center of all your sexual energy. The energy moves very close to the gonads gland. If this gland is not working properly it will create a lot of trouble, cramps and numbness in the legs and pain or disease in the reproductive areas. This all happens easily if the gonads are not working properly.

Active Symptoms:

Expression. You can express yourself well – your feelings, thoughts and emotions. You're able to express them in some way.

Not over-emotional. You don't get too stuck in your emotions that they take over you.

Strong instinct. You know what you need to do.

Fearless. You're not trapped being always scared of everything.

Healthy sex organs. You don't have any problems with sexual function at all.

Inactive Symptoms:

Unemotional. You're apathetic and don't seem to feel much.

Closed-off. You're not open with other people.

Scattered. Your mind is full of scattered thoughts and you have very little ability to focus.

Without peace. You don't feel any peace inside.

Overactive Symptoms:

Sensitive. You're easily affected by little things.

Over-emotional. Too into your emotions.

A lot of sexual energy. You have an extreme amount of sexual energy and don't know how to raise it upward to higher thinking. You can become a rapist, or abuse others sexually.

Svadhisthana's element is water. If you live near any water it will help you very much. Any time you go to the ocean, even if you are just on the sand, or by a river or a lake, any kind of water helps to open up your second chakra when you're there. If you can't visit water all the time, it will even help if you have water sounds on your phone or computer to listen to. When a person is lucky enough to live by water, they begin to open up and express what they're feeling rather than keeping it inside.

Many young people feel restless, like they are searching for something. They keep going here and there and they can never stay in one place for long, or stick to one career or opportunity. It's because their second chakras are blocked and it causes them to feel homeless, even if they have good friends and a nice place to live. They're not homeless, but their feelings are like that. They need to work on their second chakra a lot, and it will give them the feeling of ease and comfort, like they have finally arrived at their home. Otherwise, they'll have no stability at all. Svadhisthana means your own home. If something is blocking the energy here then they have to do a lot of work on it. In the Hindu sect, swamis wear the color of this chakra, but it used to be symbolic. Nowadays they don't know the meaning of it. This kind of restless feeling can take a person the wrong way in their life because they will keep pulling at many things never getting anywhere. They won't succeed in their goals, no matter how much inspiration they have. Stability in life is very important.

The two sounds for this chakra are "*vam*," and "*raakini*." They will create that energy which gets rid of your restlessness. Vam is pronounced like "lung," but with a V. All of these sounds will be like that. Same way as daakini, when you recite raakini, it needs to be very long – that is how you get the effect. Like this: raaaaaaaaaaaaaaaaaaakini. Remember you have to end the sound with "kini," the cap. Otherwise it will not work right. Recite vam for two to three minutes at the least, and recite raakini at least 108 times.

The power of this chakra is Vishnu – the preserving power, protective power and sustaining power. It means you have to think about your protection. What do you need to do to take care of yourself? You have to make sure you're going the right way, otherwise this chakra will be inactive.

The sense of the Svadhisthana chakra is the sense of taste. But there is a secret. If you go only by the taste alone, rich and tasty foods, then it doesn't work. It has a meaning. Our body needs six kinds of taste. If we don't have these tastes in our body, it will not be healthy. I call it the six *rasa*, juices. It helps to activate your Svadhistana chakra. The first rasa is sour, followed by: sweet, spicy, bitter, salty and *kshaaya*. Kshaaya is like an olive taste, that's how they call it in India. Yogic people are missing the secret of the Svadhisthana chakra; they don't know how to activate it because they get rid of all the tastes from their body. We need all these six tastes.

Sweets are cold in nature, so it's bad to eat too many of them.

Without salt the human is the most dangerous species on earth. Even if they bite a cobra, the snake will die. That is without salt. It dissolves all the poisons in our body. Everyone has some salt in their body, but it needs to be balanced with the other five tastes. Sea salt is considered good salt, but the best kind is the salt from mines, like in Africa and Pakistan. This kind of salt heals the second chakra. Don't be crazy about it – if you can't find that salt just use what you can find. Natural mine salt is best.

Bitter tastes we don't like much, but the body needs it. It's difficult to over-eat bitter things, but make sure your body has enough. Once a week is sufficient. Make some bitter juice, like natural orange juice or grapefruit juice. *Karela* is a bitter melon from India. It's extremely bitter, but like medicine.

For spice, crush red chilies and mix salt to make a sauce for eating with your bread. Or, you can cook your meals with crushed chilies sometimes.

For kshaaya, there is something from India, it's called *Triphala*: three bitter fruits mixed together. One is called harada, one is baheda and another is amvala. These are very difficult to eat. You can chew the harada and drink water. The best thing is to have equal amounts of the three fruits and grind them into a powder. Mix with water in a glass and leave it overnight to drink early in the morning. The taste is difficult but it will help. Methi seeds, are used in Indian cooking, too. In English they're called black cumin, or fenugreek seeds. Don't chew them. Soak them in water overnight and eat them early in the morning on an empty stomach. Bitter things suck out bad bacteria in the body, but also create dryness in the body if there is too much. Over-eating will create trouble for this chakra and can make your energy flow downward. Limit your intake of food or your organs can be damaged.

Herbs and spices that will help this chakra are roasted fennel seeds, red onion, sometimes raw red onion, but only a small amount, and wild garlic, not regular garlic.

If you want to try and hear the inner-sound of the Svadhisthana chakra, practice three to five minutes of Chandra Bhedi pranayama. Do the same thing for the second chakra as you did for the first chakra; sit and close your eyes; become still. You might begin to hear the sound of water trickling inside of you. It's a beautiful sound and means that your second chakra is beginning to wake up. It's like a little water fountain trickling, or a small brook.

For crystals and metals you can use citrine, moonstone, coral and amber. Aluminum, copper, iron and nickel as well.

Yoga postures to open the Svadhisthana chakra are simhasana, lion posture, siddhasana, chakrasana, and bhumananasana, the greeting earth posture. Chakrasana is with your arms and legs extended all the way lifting you up off the ground as you face upward, like a wheel. Bhekasana, the frog posture, is also good for this chakra. Try to stay in frog posture for five minutes, and when you come out of the position recite "Namo Aayariyaanam." *Yoni mudra* is the mudra that will help your second chakra. This mudra is a little more difficult and requires practice to perfect it, maybe up to six months, because of the complicated finger placement.

Aromatherapy will help if you use jasmine oil, juniper oil, rosemary oil. Any natural foods that are orange or yellowish-orange in color will make this chakra very healthy. Yellow tomatoes, tangerines, nectarines, yellow cabbage, pumpkin, apricots, peaches, oranges, papaya, carrots, mango, butternut squash, kumquat, and sweet potatoes.

Orange is the color of the Svadhisthana chakra, and it's an important color. It's the color of wisdom, it can heal your emotions, and sometimes when you have a lot of desires it can help calm them. It's a very powerful chakra make sure it's always open. Visualize orange light building up in your second chakra, bring you the feeling that you're home. Wherever you are, you are home. That is the feeling this chakra gives you when it's open. Place your right hand on your forehead, on your third-eye, and your left hand on your second chakra. Visualize all the orange light entering in you and going up your spine to the Svadhisthana.

Or, you can visualize a crimson-colored, six-petaled lotus flower. In the center of the flower is a white crescent moon, and this flower is in the water. Underneath the lotus flower, there is a crocodile, and it's actually resting on the crocodile. It's silently resting, so it seems the crocodile is carrying the flower. Crocodiles represent water, because they can stay very still like the water. All the dolphins, whales, other animals, they're always active and moving about, but the crocodile can stay very still.

Orange has many benefits. When you breathe in orange light with your breath, all the muscle spasms and cramps will begin to heal if you feel them. You have to see the light going into your body with your breath. It will increase your metabolism and give a lot of strength to the lungs. Sometimes women can't produce breast-milk when their baby is born, so this orange light will help those glands to function properly if you visualize it coming in through your breath. Orange brings a lot of ideas and mental concepts. It strengthens the emotions and your sense of well-being and cheerfulness. Orange symbolizes prosperity. If you have a cold, asthma, epilepsy, gallstones, lung conditions, tumors or mental exhaustion, orange can help all of these things to heal. Wear orange-colored clothes and sleep by orange light.

Use the solarization technique and get a glass bottle that is orange in color and fill it with water. After it sits in direct sun all day long it gets a lot of medicinal properties that can heal you on many levels. Drink it in the evening and your chakra will begin to balance. You'll feel at home and never get restless.

Many things can work to open the Svadhisthana chakra. If you have a big area of yellow and orange flowers, maybe a park or flower garden, meditate there and this chakra will come to life quickly. Sometimes if you have complete privacy you can find a spot outside where you can be naked for a few minutes, lie on your stomach and then your back so your whole body is touched by the sun. This is good for you. Early morning is the best, maybe in late spring or early summer when it is warm enough outside. In the afternoon it doesn't work as well. Practice deep breathing while in the sun here. If you try this make sure you know that no one will see you and you really have privacy. You have to always protect yourself. There is a song I wrote very long ago about Parshvanath, the first kundalini master, and two lines from it will open the second chakra:

"Jai Parshva Jai Parshva Jai Parshva devaa. Mataa jaaki vaamaa devi pitaa ashvasenaa."

Energy is coming from the Muladhara chakra, up to the Svadhisthana chakra. Sometimes it flows in as anger, ego, jealousy or other negativities. Kundalini automatically begins to flow downward in negativity. Remember that always. When you have any desire for sex it begins to flow down. You have to kick upward your sexual energy, so it goes higher to the other chakras and transforms. How do you transform your anger? You have to increase your compassion, and automatically your anger gets smaller and smaller. In the *Awakening the Soul* retreat I teach at Siddhayatan, I always say, "Whatever you focus on in your life, that becomes stronger." It is a universal law. If you focus on getting rid of your anger, it will only get stronger. It's the same way with your sexual energy. You can transform your sexual energy by seeing the result of those cravings and understanding them deeply. Every time you indulge in sexuality you lose your energy and feel weak afterward. If you're aware, you will feel those things. If you save that energy and never waste it, it builds up and begins to rise through your chakras and you feel full of energy all the time. You'll never be tired. Don't think it's a bad thing that someone has a lot of sexual energy; it means they have a chance to transform it and go higher. It depends how they use it. There are always two sides. If someone doesn't have any anger, it is very difficult to create that kind of energy to transform it and move upward. Anger is a very strong energy, and if you have a lot of it then you can transform it. But if you are more apathetic and lazy, you don't have any energy to start with, it will take much longer to create it. Sexual energy is the same. It's very strong energy and can take you higher. People just don't know how to transform it and they get stuck in it. They have to begin to raise it higher and higher, little by little, by thinking positive, thinking of how to increase their compassion, love, forgiveness and always do some kind of practical sadhana like pranayama, Purnam Yoga, mantras and meditation. That automatically begins to transform your energy. Most people try to control the energy, and it jumps even more in the wrong direction. The Catholic Church and many Hindu temples condemn sex, and tell you that if you indulge in it, you'll go to hell. They create fear, and in that fear sexual energy gets really messed up. It will never have the chance to transform if the person is in fear.

Transformation will happen when you increase your love towards everyone, the whole universe and all living beings. I can tell you the negative approach to anything, not just sex, makes your life very complicated and will take you in the wrong direction because you are flowing in negativity. If your approach is positive, it will make your life joyful and healthy and beautiful. The positive approach is to think how you can save the energy and take make yourself higher.

MANIPURA: THE THIRD CHAKRA

The third chakra is called *Manipura*. It's very important – I mentioned before that it's the axle in the body, the center of the body. If this chakra doesn't function, you're in trouble. Once the axle is broken, your life cannot go forward. "Mani" means the "jewels," or "center." "Pura," in Sanskrit, is the "stream." It means the stream of jewels; it's a hidden treasure. Some people also know it as the solar plexus, which has something to do with the sun, but no one knows this teaching anymore. The Manipura chakra is near the navel; people say that it's in the navel, but that's wrong. It's near the navel only. The pancreas is in this area, and if the energy in the Manipura is not moving properly then you'll find that your pancreas is having trouble.

Active Symptoms:

Balanced. You have balance and stay centered.

Unaffected by criticism. You can take criticism from others without reacting to it negatively.

Oneness with the universe. You feel that everything is a part of you.

Confidence. You carry yourself with confidence and don't shy from things.

In control of your own life. You are the one deciding where your life goes.

Grace and divinity. You have a sense of grace and divinity that others notice.

Inactive symptoms:

Passive. You're passive in your life and let opportunities slip from your hands.

Indecisive. You don't have the ability to make up your mind.

Overactive Symptom:

Aggressive. You are over-aggressive and others notice it often.

Fire is the element of the Manipura. In the winter if you sit near a fire, this chakra gets some energy from it and becomes more active. Fire is important for this chakra, because it helps your digestive system burn everything. It doesn't get stuck when there is fire. If you hear roaring fire it will help tremendously, too. Even if you can't be near the fire, you can find the sound of fire somewhere to listen to on your computer or phone.

For this chakra, recite the sounds "raṁ" and "laakini." Raṁ is pronounced like you're saying, "lung," with an R. Recite this sound for at least two to three minutes to get the results. If you practice these sounds every day it will help you a lot. Even if you're sitting on a bench in the park you can just do them and it's quick. You can be anywhere. Laakini is very powerful, and remember it has to be said long, about five to ten seconds. Laaaaaaaaaaaaaaaaaaaaaaaaaaaaaaaaaaaaaakini. Always remember the cap at the end to keep the energy in the right place.

Manipura is ruled by the third power of God, Rudra. It's the destructive power of God. In Indian mythology they call it Shiva. God doesn't destroy you, only your lower qualities like anger, ego, jealousy, and so on. Think about this.

The Manipura is the center of our body and it's very important. Like a bicycle, all the spokes are connected with the axle, and in the same way, all the chakras are connected with the Manipura. It has a lot of secrets about it. We disconnect the silver-cord when we're born and after that we have to breathe and eat to survive. As soon as the baby is born, the cord is cut and they cry for the first time. They feel like they are taken away from heaven. The parents become so happy because they see their child is alive. They're not crying because they're alive, they are crying because they now have to breathe and work. It's called effort. Any time you have to create effort, stress begins. Stress comes first into the Manipura chakra and it's messed up more than the other chakras. Many kids have jaundice and other diseases, they can't digest food right away, they become very stressed out. It's because they feel so much stress from having to put efforts to survive and live. When the energy here is really messed up, the child can have ADD or ADHD – Attention Deficit Disorder, and Attention Deficit Hyperactivity Disorder. They cannot sit still at all and if they want to do something they can't focus on it. Have you ever noticed people sitting on a chair and they keep shaking their legs or feet or moving their fingers? Why do they do it? Their third chakra is not balanced and there is some kind of stress in them. They don't even know it. Since their birth they have felt that stress of being taken from the womb and having to put their own effort to eat, to breathe, to drink and to survive. Maybe they don't know where it comes from, but deep down it's there. It's the stress from putting effort and it can really create a lot of problems, especially in children. The pills and medicines don't do much to help it. They need to have the right guidance so they can straighten out their energy.

The sense of this chakra is very powerful; it can do a lot of damage to you, but it can help you also. The sense is sight. And there is a big secret about it. Our eyes are the most sensitive part of our body. Somehow, all the tension is held in the eyes. People complain about pain in their shoulders, their back, legs; it's all related to the eyes. The first thing we connect with is outer objects, seen with our eyes. Even more than the ears. Our eyes hold so much stress in them, and all of that stress flows to the navel and our Manipura becomes very weak. So, instead of breathing the proper way, through our stomach like a baby does, we start to breathe through our chests and it invites all the illness. A lot of trouble is created by our sight. Did you ever notice that sometimes when women are holding a lot of tension and they begin to cry, they feel better afterward? Women don't have heart attacks as much as men do, because they release some tension. In society today, men are taught not to cry, that it's a sign of weakness. These ideas need to stop. Crying does not show weakness. It helps to relieve some of the stress in our system, even if it is only temporary. The stress is not gone forever. It helps the Manipura just for a little while. I mentioned earlier about the ancient technique called tratka. People are confused that all of these techniques are coming from the *Yoga Sutras*, but Patañjali was not really the author. He simply collected the information and put it together to share with people. Parshvanath was the one giving all the teachings at that time. He taught about tratka, and this is the real permanent solution to release all the stress from this chakra. What's taken in by the eyes has to be released by the eyes.

When you practice tratka, what begins to happen after you don't blink for some time? All the tension from every part of your body will come into your head, and your eyes begin to tear. Tears will fall down your cheeks and this gives you the permanent relief. Once the tension leaves, it is gone forever. Unless you invite it back again, that is a different story. But how many will even practice? When your eyes are fully open and you concentrate on the black circle, all the thoughts begin to disappear. As soon as you will blink all the thoughts come back into you. But when they're absent, that is the time God is waiting to enter into you. Kundalini is waiting for you to be in the thoughtless state. Instead of creating the time, you choose to hold all the tension and pollution in your body and you expect your energy to rise? Wake up. Remove your tension and remove your stress. Practice tratka every day. It's a practical technique, and you can see the results right away. If you have glaucoma then it is not safe for you to practice.

For crystals, you can use gold topaz or citrine, and tiger's eye is the best for the Manipura.

Kapalbhati pranayama is the breathing exercise you need to do in order to hear the sound of the Manipura. Try to disconnect from your senses. Maybe in the beginning you will have to close your ears, but after practice you won't have to do it anymore. You'll be able to disconnect from your whole body even. Suddenly you'll hear a faint sound, like bagpipes in the distance.

Practicing the suryanamaskara sequence of yoga postures will help this chakra to balance. Suryanamaskara is the "sun salutation," which is a combination of about twelve postures and it floods your body with energy. You can also do simhasana and kurmasana, lion and tortoise postures. In the Jain teachings it's written that Jain monks and nuns have to control their senses like the tortoise, keeping all their limbs inside their shell and they're protected. But Jains misunderstood it fully. It's the system of how to activate this chakra, but they took the literal meaning and didn't try to think about it. The signs are there; it means you have to let go of all your senses. Nothing comes to you, no thoughts, nothing. All the senses stop bothering you. It's simple but they misunderstood it. The technique comes from Tirthankara Shri Parshvanath.

The best posture for the Manipura is mayurasana, the peacock. If someone is able to do it perfectly, and they accidentally take in poison in their food or some other way, they can digest the poison fully with this posture. Years ago in India, a popular Jain Acharya tried to poison and kill me out of jealousy. I knew he put poison in my food, but I still ate it. Then right after eating I went into peacock posture to rid the poison out of my body. He was shocked when he saw me hours later and couldn't believe that the poison didn't work. Decades later, he died of poisoning; a Jain nun poisoned him. Anyone that tries to kill a master will collect tremendous bad karma. What I am sharing with you here in this book works. You just need to practice it. Peacock creates incredible fire in the navel. Seek the truth, don't just believe in it. You've been believing for centuries and thousands of years that there is a God, but it's time to wake up. Find what God is for yourself. The truth is in you. Mani means jewel, and you have the diamond in you. This chakra is the axle in the body and you have the super-instrument that even angels wish to have. Without this human instrument, the soul cannot be liberated. Other postures you can do are dandasana, staff posture, and nauvasana, the boat posture. These strengthen the navel center a lot. *Nabhi*, in Sanskrit, also means navel

These postures will vibrate the nabhi. The nabhi is the center that is very important. You need the navel to be hit hard to vibrate it. If you become a master in tortoise posture and peacock posture you will really help yourself. Another posture is hastapandugasana, standing forward-bend, which is when you do a forward-bend to catch your toes with your fingers. It creates a lot of energy in the Manipura and it opens right away. *Matangi mudra* will open the third chakra if you do it all the time.

This chakra has many other secrets. We were connected with the mother when we were born. We were connected to the absolute. Like the baby is connected by the silver-cord to the mother; the mother eats and so does the baby, the mother breathes and so does the baby. It's a natural connection. When that cord is disconnected the baby will cry. We are seeking that comfort again, that connection. The baby cries when it's born because it has to try and survive now. Before it didn't have to do anything, it was relaxed, and now it is in the world and receives stress from everywhere. This silver-cord is symbolic. You can be connected with God, with soul, but you need to know the sound and nobody teaches it. You have to say it very loud. If you recite the sound "*saahu,*" it will shake this center so much. It has to be very loud to get this result. You say it like this: saaaaaaaaaaaaaaaa-hu! The "hu" has to be full of force and very loud. Your stomach will shoot in when you say it, because all of your breath is exhaled by the force and that hits the navel and causes a big vibration there. Recite it 108 times and begin to imagine the silver-cord is being created again. It will connect you with God directly. You will feel a lot of energy and heat.

"*Arhum,*" is a beautiful sound. It is the name of God – Brahma, absolute. If you want to remember what absolute is, recite, "arhum." It's the same meaning as the Namokar mantra, because everything is included in arhum. It represents everyone; from the person on the spiritual path, to the spiritual teachers, enlightened persons and finally the liberated souls. There's a science in it. It's the seed of the Siddhas. They all have a name in their last body, but after that when they merge you can remember all of them at the same time with this sound, "arhum." It represents all the Siddhas and becomes the seed mantra for them. You can be in tune with God by reciting this mantra and it will protect you. It creates fire in you, the energy of the Siddhas; when it represents them it means it creates that energy.

For aromatherapy you can use lemon, rosemary and juniper to activate your third chakra.

To increase the energy in the Manipura, make sure you're eating yellow-skinned fruits and vegetables: apricots, carrots, cantaloupe, corn, yellow peppers, yellow lentils, grapefruit, mango, melon, pineapple, yellow onion, plantains, passion fruit, star fruit, peaches, squash, and turnips. Butter can help if it isn't eaten in excess, or have many added ingredients to it. It has to be more pure, like ghee, clarified butter. Eat at the right time when your chakra is open. If your Pingala nadi is not open, it's better not to eat because it won't be digested; the fire is not working in your body at that time. There is a way to open it though. If you notice only your Ida nadi is open, the left nostril and known as the moon channel for its cooling effects on the body, then you can lie down on your right side and try to be relaxed. Breathe slow and deeply, but don't force this breath. After two or three minutes both of the nadis will be more balanced and you'll be able to digest your meal. If only the Ida nadi is open then you can only digest liquids. If only the Pingala nadi is open then you can only digest more solid foods.

Why do they call this the solar plexus? The sun works with this chakra like a lotus flower. When the sun rises, the lotus flower blossoms and its petals begin to open fully, but when the sun sets the lotus flower's petals begin to close. Same thing, when the sun is close to us this chakra is always open. Whatever you eat will digest when the sun is close. After the sun sets and moves away from us, food doesn't digest in our stomachs. If you eat something heavy it will sit in your stomach all night and create trouble for your intestines, so I don't suggest eating later after sunset. The best thing to do is make sure you eat dinner within 90 minutes of the sun going down. Because after 90 minutes the chakra is still open half-way and can digest a meal, but if you wait longer to eat it will have difficulty. After three hours the Manipura is fully closed. So, if the sun sets at 7pm, the chakra will be half-way closed at 8:30pm, and fully closed at 10pm. In the morning it is a little different; when the sun begins to rise, it is already open half-way. It's all the way open 90 minutes after sunrise. In the Jain religion, the monks and nuns do not eat before sunrise or after sunset. The tradition started partly because in those days there was no lighting system to help people see in the dark. The way people lived, their homes had simple windows with no glass or coverings, and many insects can come inside freely. If the monks and nuns went to get food at this time, there was a chance they might eat a living being if they happened to fall in the food without being seen. The true meaning behind this discipline, which they lost, was that eating in the dark with a closed third chakra will cause a lot of trouble in the body.

This is a big secret about this chakra, because you can keep your body in the best health and always feel light. It's best to eat a very light breakfast, especially if you eat around sunrise, and eat the heaviest meal for lunch so there is plenty of energy to digest the food. For dinner, eat a meal that is less heavy; not too much bread or heavy beans. Don't sleep until two to three hours after eating your last meal. That way your body is still awake to digest. I often say there is a simple reason why Jesus, Mahavira, Buddha and Krishna had such attractive personalities. The reason is because they knew when to eat and when to drink. If you eat when you are not really hungry, it's unhealthy. After having the meal you will feel heavy and uneasy. But the person who knows how to eat and drink, they will still feel light and joyful after a meal. I suggest when your Pingala nadi is blocked, the right nostril, it's better not to eat a full meal and have more liquid instead. When you are really breathing in the Sushumna nadi, you don't feel hunger or thirst at all, so breathing that way is more important, because you will eat only when your body feels real hunger.

The morning is a beautiful time of day and has many secrets about it. In India it is called *Brahma muhurta*, the Godly time. Tremendous amounts of oxygen are produced by the trees at this time, 90 minutes before sunrise, and it's a very quiet time of day. Most people are sleeping then so the atmosphere is not crowded with all the thoughts throughout the day. I always recommend for people to sit in the fresh air before the sunrise and take deep breaths. You gain so much energy from it and will feel fresh and positive throughout the day. If you practice pranayama techniques during Godly time it will be even better for you. If you can't be outside, even just open a window to get a little fresh air in the room, or bundle up if it's cold. Your entire day will be transformed. Make sure you are up early because there is more oxygen 90 minutes before the sunrise, and it slowly gets less and less. Then later in the day when the sun sets, trees start producing carbon dioxide, so avoid doing intensive breathing at that time.

Breathing in yellow color helps a lot for the Manipura chakra. It generates energy into the muscles and they become very strong. This is the best color to strengthen your nervous system and brain. It carries positive magnetic currents that will strengthen the nervous system automatically. The brain is reached by the nervous system, so if a person's nervous system is not working properly, the brain can suddenly slow down as well. When they slow down they cannot think right. They try to think positive, but suddenly negative thoughts will enter. It helps the liver, the intestines and the skin, too – your skin will become very soft. If you do it, you will feel it. Yellow is the color of intellect and gives you good perception. Perception is different from logic – logic is just illusion. You perceive the real things. Yellow light heals constipation, and diabetes will be weakened with this color. It heals a lot of gastric problems, too. Mental depression can be turned around. The Manipura needs to be straightened out or there will be a lot of blockages in the aspect of intelligence. It brings a lot of reasoning to a person. When there are many problems with this chakra they won't perceive the things they're supposed to.

From the Namokar mantra, there is one line that creates the yellow color throughout the body. The third line, "Namo Aayariyaanaṁ," is what you need to recite. When you pronounce it, it's like this: nah-mo eye-ya-ree-yaa-nung. All the yellow light will suddenly flood your body and begins to heal you. The way the vowels are combined in this sound does this automatically. Recite it more and more to create tremendous light and heal the Manipura chakra.

One of the strongest techniques for balancing the chakras is the solarization technique. It's very strong, and the Manipura chakra needs to be hit strongly. Make sure you can find a glass bottle that's yellow. After you fill it with water, remember to place it where it will receive direct sunlight all day. It can't be in the shade at all. From sunrise to sunset, when it sits for this long in the sunlight it gets so much energy from the sun which is transformed by the colored glass and energizes the water. With this technique you can really help your center, your axle.

Don't forget that this chakra is the most important. All of the chakras are important, but the Manipura is special because it's your center. You need to breathe and live from your center. This way you can always remain balanced, and nothing will affect you. That's how you'll find peace, and achieve your goal of liberation.

ANAAHAT: THE FOURTH CHAKRA

Each chakra has a different function, creates different energy and affects our mind and bodies differently. The fourth chakra is very important for the human life. It's the first step towards God, towards the higher power. All the power begins in your heart, not at the lower chakra. The first three chakras are considered the lower part of the body. The fourth chakra, also known as the heart chakra, is called *Anaahat*. It's important because all the emotions like love, helping others, compassion, forgiveness, kindness, all the things you talk about, they all reside in the heart. "Ana" means "no," and "ahat" means "sound." It's soundless. Even though the name of this chakra means soundless, it is the trouble-maker, because of our relations with other people.

Our hearts become hurt by many things, and other people don't really understand what we are feeling, so the heart gets hit deeply. In Sanskrit, Anaahat also means that it hits you. All the emotions hit you deeply, so you have to be careful about this chakra, because if it's not balanced you can go down emotionally and it's hard to get out. I always tell people that when the heart chakra works in you, then you are very close to God. Because this chakra is soundless. It's a saying that God lives in your heart, but remember God lives in your heart only if it's pure like a child is, innocent and divine. Babies are born with a pure heart. That is the kind of heart you need to have. God wants to enter in you, to penetrate into your heart, but there is no space because of the mess from all of your emotions. One poet said, "The picture of my beloved is hidden in my heart. Whenever I want to see it, I have to bow my head down." What does it mean? Bowing down means you have to crush your ego. God is not far away from you; it's the closest thing to you. Make your heart as pure as possible. If your heart is not pure, then the mystery of God is far away from you. It can be revealed to you, but you have to open your heart that way. If not, you will never understand who you really are. You'll wander in emotions and they may lead you elsewhere. This is why the heart chakra is very important.

Active Symptoms:

Caring. You care about others and think of what they need.

Unconditional love. You have the feeling of love towards everyone and everything, with no expectations.

Brotherhood. Do you think about it, or have the feeling? We are all on the same route, no matter where we come from. We have the same blood, drink the same water, laugh and cry the same way.

Compassion. Not only to your friends or family, but to all of the animal kingdom, little bugs, all people, plants, the whole earth.

Devotion. Maybe you are devoted to your work, or your family or your country. Real devotion is where love ends. It means devotion is on the higher level.

Spiritual growth. Are you working on improving yourself and awakening your soul?

Good relations. Do you keep good relations with all the people you meet?

Inactive Symptoms:

Cold and unfriendly. You're not warm or welcoming at all to others.

Overactive Symptoms:

Selfishness. You do things for yourself without thinking of how to help those around you.

Too much love. You begin to suffocate others with how much love you show to others.

The Anaahat chakra's element is the air, so you need to make sure you are breathing the right way. Learn to breathe like a baby does, the natural way. They never breathe from their chest, always from their belly. Watch a baby when they are sleeping and you'll see that their belly goes up and down. If you can go outside during the 90 minutes before sunrise and breath very deeply to bring pure oxygen into your system. This balances the heart chakra very much. You will be fresh all day long. You can also listen to the sounds of wind on a recording; that will help a lot, too.

The sounds which will helps the heart chakra vibrate more are "yam" and "kaakini." You already know how to pronounce them: yam is like the English word "young," and kaakini has to be with a long, extended breath. Kaaaaaaaaaaaaaaaaaakini. Don't just say these sounds quickly, they must be very long. Recite yam for two to three minutes and kaakini recite 108 times. You can feel the change in you suddenly, but you need to first build up strength in the practice by reciting very often. There is another sound in the Namokar mantra that creates the green energy in your body and helps the heart a lot. "Namo Uvajjhaayanam." Pronounced like this: nah-mo oo-vuh-jai-aa-nung. It automatically creates dark green light and opens your heart as soon as you begin reciting it. There is a very old sutra written in Prakrit about Parshvanath called the *Uvasaggaharam Stotram*. There are five verses in it, and if you can recite this sutra 25 times, even just once a week, the chakra begins to work so quickly you won't believe it. The sounds create a lot of energy.

Uvasaggaharam pasam, pasam vandami kamma-ghan-mukkam;
Visahar-vis-ninnasam, mangal kallan avasam. 1
Visahar-fuling mantam, kanthe dharei jo saya manuo;
Tassa gah rog mari, duttha-jara janti uvasamam. 2
Chitthau dure manto, tujza panamo vi bahu-falo hoi;
Naratiriesu vi jiva, pavanti na dukkha-dohaagam. 3
Tuha sammatte laddhe, chintamani kappa-payavabbhahie;
Pavanti avigghenam, jiva ayaramaram thanam. 4
Ea santhuo mahayas, bhatti-bbhar-nibbharen hiyaenam;
Ta dev dijza bohim, bhave bhave pas jinachanda. 5

Isha is what rules this chakra. "Isha" means "lord," or "God." It means that if you keep your heart very pure then God is in your heart, so make sure to purify your heart. I guarantee God is not far away from you.

The sense that belongs to the Anaahat, the heart chakra, is touch. It means that if the heart chakra becomes active, you're not too emotional or a kind of touchy person. If it's overactive you become too touchy and emotional. Your heart is open but it's too open. It brings you the wrong messages. It's better to have knowledge about the senses of the chakras. The sense is touch, so don't be too close to people and be touching them all the time, or you will get the wrong messages because of the energy in your heart, and you can be affected by it too much. You bring emotions into you through the touch, and it can hurt you if you get the wrong message. Like people who are always hugging and touching, kissing their friends, hugging babies, holding hands – sometimes it can be too much energy and cause a lot of chaos in a person's heart if it's overactive. It means to be aware of touch and it will help your Anaahat chakra to be balanced more.

For crystals you can use emerald and green jade. If you touch the emerald on your heart for a few minutes or wear it in a necklace it will do a lot of good. Men can have emerald on a ring if they don't want to wear it around their neck.

The heart chakra really opens when you practice the yoga postures bhujanghasana, the cobra posture, ardha matsyendrasana, half-fish posture, matsyasana, full-fish posture and ustrasana, camel posture. While in the fish postures, practice Kapalbhati pranayama and it will clean the pollution out from your heart. When you become established in the camel posture, what you can do is go deep into yourself and close your eyes. Try to let go and enter into a meditative state. When you master any posture, stay in it for two to five minutes and it will begin creating the certain energy in your body. After staying in ustrasana for a while, you'll hear there is nothing around you, and all you can hear is the inner-sound of chimes coming from within you. When you really are in meditation you begin to hear these sounds, but you have to be fully there. It cannot be created, it can only happen. Sit and gaze at the tip of your nose with half-open eyes. This will take you into the Sushumna nadi, into your heart, right away. It takes practice because you can sometimes get a small headache in the beginning, but keep your practice going and you'll be surprised. By practicing the *Padma mudra*, you can activate the heart chakra.

To hear the inner-sound, practice Anulom Vilom pranayama for five minutes, and close all your senses to hear the sound of the fourth chakra, the heart chakra. Forget everything. When you go deep you'll begin hearing the sound of bells and chimes. Like very long and drawn out chiming sounds.

Aromatherapy can help your heart chakra through sandalwood, cedar wood and rose.

Your heart needs the color green in order to open up. You can create that light in you by eating green fruits and vegetables. Cucumbers, zucchini, green grapes, spinach, okra, karela, the bitter Indian melon, green apples, green tomatoes, artichoke, basil, arugula, avocado, kale, broccoli, kiwi, Chinese cabbage, honeydew melon, jalapeño and poblano peppers, cilantro, lettuce, swiss char, methi herb. Methi herb opens the chakra a lot. It's similar to cilantro but in India it's mixed with potato and brings a lot of warmness in the heart and can heal many diseases. Saffron, too, if you mix it with rice. Remember to cook items like kale and spinach. Do not eat them raw. They contain a lot of bacteria, so it is best to cook them instead.

Visualize green light near your heart to balance this chakra. The Anaahat chakra is between the thymus gland and the heart. Visualize all the green color coming into your third-eye and going down to your heart.

Breathing in, visualize all the green light surrounding your heart and filling it. Your chakra begins to balance itself out. All you have to do is visualize the color. Visualize a smokey-blue lotus flower with 12 petals. In the center of the flower is a white triangle and a blue triangle that form a star together. This image will open up the heart and balance it. If energy is not moving in the Anaahat chakra, the thymus gland and thyroid gland will be affected a lot. They won't function well. If you have any kind of heart ache or heart pains, you need to think that the energy isn't moving properly so you have to work on balancing your heart chakra. Otherwise it will be weak and you can have a heart attack. Liver and lungs are affected by this chakra as well. This chakra can help keep you alive – if you have a clot in your blood, then it won't circulate well and you can become very sick. Maybe you won't have a long life. It's very dangerous to have a clot in your blood. Green has a lot of good effects on the body. It's soothing, cooling and calming – physically, mentally and emotionally. It can relieve tension in the blood vessels. When the blood vessels are tense you can't think the right way. Automatically the blood pressure is lowered when the heart chakra is balanced. Green can make a person very warm. Sometimes you can be very down emotionally, and green will make you warm and bring you up from the lowness. It stimulates the pituitary gland near the Ajna chakra, the third-eye, and helps to build muscle and tissue. Wear green clothing and sleep near green light. An important benefit of the green color is that it loosens and balances the etheric body – the astral body – and when the astral body is healthy you will have positive thinking and dreams. When you wake up in the morning you'll feel clear and joyful. It's the color of fertility and new life. If you want to feel young forever then visualize green light. It can heal asthma, heart problems, high blood pressure, mental irritation, reduces malaria and helps with sleeping problems. If you need to strengthen your respiratory system then green light will do a very good job. It brings so much strength into the respiratory system. You can even use a green light and lay under it for a while. This will help.

You know the solarization technique now, so find a dark green glass bottle, and let it sit in the sun all day with water inside. This will heal your heart and bring those higher qualities into you.

The path resides only in the pure heart. Remember this always. It cannot stay in a heart that is polluted by so many emotions. Work hard to continue dissolving these lower-qualities by doing your sadhana. One day your heart will be fully clean and you'll feel that the entire universe is a part of you, and you a part of it. That is the deeper love that is beyond feelings and thoughts.

VISHUDDHI: THE FIFTH CHAKRA

Vishuddhi is the name of the fifth chakra; the throat chakra. It's considered a higher chakra, because from the Anaahat upwards, these chakras take you into spirituality. The Vishuddhi is between the thyroid and thymus gland in your throat. This chakra brings you the ability to express and communicate very well. In Sanskrit, "Vishuddhi" means "purification." You have to purify this chakra if you want to communicate in your life, share your ideas with the world. If you have a sore throat often, or sore upper-arms, then you need to check on the thyroid and thymus glands and see how they're doing. It indicates the energy in your Vishuddhi chakra is not working right.

Active Symptoms:

Good expression. You can put your thoughts into words very clearly.

Communication. People can understand you well when you communicate.

Creativity. Are you creative in all aspects or just one thing? Spread your creativity.

Hear the inner-voice. This isn't like you hear God talking to you. It means you can hear yourself, what you know on the inside.

Inactive Symptoms:

Inability to speak. You can't speak at all, or have a lot of trouble speaking.

Shyness. Too much shyness is not a good thing.

No expression of thoughts. You often fail to express your thoughts.

Overactive Symptoms:

Speak too much. It can irritate other people and they may think you are annoying, but you don't notice.

Lack of listening skills. You cannot listen very well, you don't hear the right message, or your heart is not in listening to others.

Bone is the element for the Vishuddhi chakra. Some people are big-boned, or even some animals are, too, such as elephants. If you know any person with big bones, it can help your chakra a lot to sit near them for ten or twenty minutes. The chakra will automatically begin to open and you're not even doing anything. People born with big bones have very little chances that their fifth chakra will be blocked or inactive.

"Haṁ" and "shaakini" are the sounds that need to be recited for the vibrations to affect the Vishuddhi. When you recite haṁ, if you place one of your hands lightly over your throat you can feel where the vibration is the most. This is the location of your chakra. It sounds like "hung" when you are reciting it the proper way. Practice it for at least two to three minutes. It works when you recite shaakini, too, if you put your hand on your throat. It's just a simple way for you to feel the vibration and find exactly where the energy is. Remember, the chakra is just an area where energy is moving in you. It is not a physical thing like a bone or tissue. It just indicates where the energy is. Recite shaakini 108 times; it opens up right away with this sound, it's so powerful. Shaaaaaaaaaaaaaaaaaakini. Like the Anaahat chakra, if you recite "Namo Uvajjhaayanaṁ," it creates also a blue light that helps the Vishuddhi chakra. One mantra that was popular in Parshvanath's time was, "*Asi Aau Sa Namaha.*" It's pronounced like this: uh-see aa-oo suh nah-muh-ha. People were always reciting this mantra. Another mantra that helps a lot is "*Aum Hriṁ Shriṁ Kliṁ Arhum Haṁsa,*" pronounced as, aum hreeng shreeng kleeng eye-ray-hung hung-suh.

The Vishuddhi chakra is ruled by Ardhnarishwar. It's a representation of God; half-male and half-female. In India they found one statue like this that's very old. All the upper chakras are ruled by God. People didn't understand what this statue was when they found it, but it's the concept of God. In those days people were very advanced, and they considered that God was not only a father, but a mother, too. Somebody made this statue so people would see it and understand. If God is only a father how can he create everything? It needs to be a mother, too. You can say either. The statue of Ardhnarishwar is very symbolic. It tells the concept of what people use to believe in that civilization. We are very backward these days.

Sound is the sense of this chakra. Sound means speech, your tongue. It's the power of speaking, and if you want to speak very well you have to work on this chakra. If you can speak clearly, all the people will understand your vision, your ideas and what you are trying to share. It can change your life and connect you with many people. Many things can help you to acquire this ability. You just need to practice these techniques that I'm sharing from Parshvanath's system.

One way is to use turquoise, sapphire and topaz, but only blue topaz. Lapis also works. These stones will heal this chakra if you hold them against your throat gently, for a few minutes.

Practice Nadi Shodhan pranayama for three minutes at least, to hear the sound of the fifth chakra. Close your ears and senses and body. Let your mind go still and quiet. The inner-sound of this chakra is like wind blowing through the trees. Or, like there is no rain but you can hear streaming water quietly. They are similar sounds.

To open this chakra, you have to open and extend your throat a lot. These are yoga postures which will help you to do so: shalabhasana, locust posture, halasana, plow posture, chakrasana, wheel posture, and ustrasana, camel posture. Ustrasana helps the Vishuddhi chakra as well, because of the intense stretch along your neck. When you master these postures your throat chakra will be cleared very quickly. Stay in them for two to five minutes, and you won't fail in communication or expression ever again in your life. To activate your Vishuddhi chakra using a mudra, practice the *Shuni mudra,* by touching the tip of your middle finger to the tip of your thumb. This mudra is known as the "seal of patience."

Aromatherapy that will help to open this chakra is lavender flower. If you can have this fragrance around you, the Vishuddhi will be more balanced while you use the other techniques to create more strength in it.

Find light foods which are naturally blue in color, such as blueberries and concord grapes. Acai is also very good for this chakra. It is close to blue so it will give the same energy.

The color belonging to this chakra's energy is light blue. Visualize it in your throat and you'll see the Vishuddhi begins to heal after some time. Our body needs a lot of blue in it. When you lack blue in your body, your metabolism is very weak. Blue increases the metabolism and your pranic-force will become so strong. It creates harmony because you become balanced, and it reduces nervous excitement. People who are over-excited can feel a lot of peace if they visualize the blue color in them. When you are going through some kind of strong emotional experience, I suggest visualizing blue, because it will help you calm down and go through the experience peacefully. Meditate where there is blue – a blue room, blue painted walls, blue light or on a blue blanket. It's the color of truth and devotion, sincerity and calmness. If you're not sincere no one will trust you. It creates intuition and higher abilities in the brain. If you will inhale it through your breath, it can help to heal chicken pox, reduce cholera and get rid of diarrhea. Eye inflammation, epilepsy, itching, insomnia, jaundice and polio can all be helped tremendously by the blue color. The more you do it, the more the chakra will heal and balance. Your energy will become very compassionate, loving, creative and communicative. Inner wisdom comes to you then. These are all brought by the blue color. Some people don't know how to speak or have a lot of mood swings and get hiccups often. This kind of light blue, while breathing it in, will help these things. It will reduce mood swings.

Find a blue glass bottle, and let it sit in the sun all day with water inside. Drink it in the evening and continue doing it each day that the sun is out.

In one aspect, the Vishuddhi chakra is the most important for health in the physical body. Many diseases can form in the body without the energy moving here. For twenty-four hours we are swallowing saliva. All day; we never stop swallowing saliva. When we eat, the saliva mixes with the food to break it apart so it can digest quickly in our intestines. You have to chew your food very well, otherwise the intestines require more energy and have more difficulty trying to break the food apart. It hurts the intestines and makes them weak over time. When you chew well it becomes a good acid and your body doesn't have to do much work.

This saliva is flowing in your body everywhere, and we don't have any control over it. Sometimes it can go too much to one place and cause problems for us. For example, when saliva flows too much into your bones, they begin to get arthritis and it will be very painful. Arthritis is difficult to heal. How can you divert this acid so it doesn't flow in one place too much? Sometimes it can go to your teeth, or ears or your eyes. You can lose sight, lose teeth and have hearing loss. You can't control it unless you know the system. Parshvanath used to teach about it. The best thing to do is change the course of this acid created by your saliva so it flows to your hair; hair doesn't have a function in your body. It turns your hair grey or white, and in society, you find that most people don't like this. If you're a teenager and your hair turns grey or white, you are very lucky, but instead you become depressed. It means the acid is already flowing to the right place, and it won't hurt your body later on. If you can learn halasana, the plow posture, and become a master in it, you have to stay here for ten to fifteen minutes. It sends all this acid to your hair. And shalabhasana, the locust posture. Your body becomes long and skinny like a humming bird. It might take you six months to divert the energy, but if you don't put effort then it won't go anywhere. It's up to you. You need to learn either or both of these postures. It will begin helping right away with hearing loss, loss of vision and things like this.

I'm bringing to life all of these teachings that came from Parshvanath.

He was the first kundalini master, and most popular Tirthankara in the Jain system. When the chakras are fully active and clear you won't have any problems in your body or mind. Sit in meditation and forget yourself. Go into *shunya*; it means nothing is there. In this situation, the thoughtless state, the chakras create so much energy and suddenly open right up.

AJNA: THE SIXTH CHAKRA

The human body contains many energy centers, but there are seven main ones. These are the chakras, and the energy moves in these places like a wheel. The sixth chakra is called the *Ajna* chakra. Ajna is the center of wisdom, real wisdom. Ajna is between the eyebrows, and people also call it the third-eye. This is the most popular chakra. The pituitary gland is the closest gland here, so you can see how well the energy is moving by checking on the health of the pituitary. Even if this chakra works thirty to forty-percent you're very lucky. This gives you a lot of inner-vision. But, if it works more than fifty or sixty-percent, then you are really lucky. That is difficult. If you find any of these symptoms in you, then you need to work to balance this chakra.

First is the spine. If the whole spine has a problem it's because the pituitary is causing it. The lower brain doesn't function well, because the pituitary gland is in the lower portion of the brain. It can create memory loss in you. It will affect the nose too; sometimes the nose is crooked. The person thinks they were born with it like that – no, it becomes crooked later on. When the nose is crooked it means something is wrong in the pituitary gland. The Ajna chakra is not open much. If the left eye loses any vision, it means this chakra is not healthy. If your hearing has problems, like you hear less and less throughout your life, it is affected by the pituitary gland.

It's important to understand, because this gland is in our heads, and remember what I said: the human is like an upside-down tree. Our roots are in our head, and we need to work on the head a lot. If someone works on their head, just the head, they can improve spiritually, but if their head is messed up, then they can be deep in illusion no matter what they're doing. They will stay in the dark, even if they believe they are not there. This chakra has to function to get out of illusion. It's the third-eye. The two physical eyes can see just the outside things, but the third-eye can see inner things. If your two eyes are closed and your third-eye is open, you can see the universe. Then you'll begin to see that the universe is not what you thought. There are millions of galaxies and even one is so big it's almost never-ending. In Sanskrit, the universe is called *Brahmanda* – infinite. It's endless. Can you imagine, in this Brahmanda, our planet is nowhere. If we make a map of the universe, this earth is not even the tiniest dot on the entire map. Where do you exist? It's just a little thing. So, why be egoistic? Why hoard all of your problems and make suffering for yourself? You need to clear your head. Work on this chakra, and that will give you power to see inside. There is infinite knowing inside of you. When this chakra is fully working, all your inner things are open and you begin to see through the stars. If you want to meditate, if you want to relax, you have to close these two eyes and go deep into your third-eye. The third-eye will take you deep into your consciousness. It's very deep – deeper than the whole ocean. Consciousness is the universe. If your consciousness is open, if your soul is open, you are everywhere then.

Active Symptoms:

Wisdom. Do you have wisdom? If you have real wisdom, you'll never make a mistake in your whole life. Wisdom is the highest point.

Intellect. Are you intelligent? Do you make an effort to learn and educate yourself?

Clairvoyance. If something comes to you, you glimpse the truth, then you are experiencing clairvoyance.

Willpower. Do you have strength and resolve in your decisions?

Visualization. Can you visualize things? Visualization is close to actualization. It's not in imagination.

Spiritual awakening. Is it happening to you? It means you're taking the step towards the path. The step is towards nonviolence. You feel oneness with all living beings, and if you feel that, then you cannot harm any one of them. You cannot eat them or kill them.

Inactive Symptoms:

Cannot think for yourself. Can you make decisions for yourself, what you want to do or not want to do? Or do you rely on others to make decisions and be told what to do?

Confusion. There is a lack of clarity and a lot of doubt.

Overactive Symptoms:

Over-imaginative. Imagination is very good, but you have to grounded at the same time.

Daydream too much. Daydreaming is also good, but are you lost in it? Do you wish for things in your life but cannot make them happen?

Hallucinations. You see things that are not there.

The element of the Ajna chakra is the subtle bodies. This physical body is a house for them. Subtle bodies are the real bodies. There is a science to it. If you look into your subtle bodies you'll be surprised to see that they are handling everything. When you're fully relaxed the bodies go out of your physical body. When you're asleep your body is fully relaxed, but when you're awake you can't do it. There is tension. That's why you have dreams when you sleep, because your subtle bodies are out of your physical body because of the relaxed state you're in, and they travel through the universe and you see what they do as a vision, as a dream. You really go to those places in your sleep. Everything looks beautiful from far away, but if you go deep into it, you know what it is. Go deep into your own body, and what will you find there? Go deep into your senses and what will you find there? If there is no skin on the top, can you believe that you wouldn't be able to stand your own body? It's full of smell. The skin keeps everything inside. Layers upon layers covering this marrow, bones and everything else. Just think about what if it wasn't there, what's going to happen? You begin to see yourself deeper and deeper. It's called *sharir preksha*. It means you begin to see your own body. The more you go and travel into it, you become so aware right away. "Why am I carrying this? Why can't I use it?" you begin to think. So, sometimes it happens, by looking at their own body people can become enlightened. It is very rare, but it happens. It depends on the person, if that is their time. It happened with one king, and he happened to be the most handsome king in that time. He was a king when it happened, and after going so deep into his body and seeing what it really is, he no longer lived in the kingdom. He was enlightened.

There are a lot of things to know, but you need to go through your own experience, go through your own body. Then, if you go through it, those particles which are around you, filling the whole universe, they are subtler than the subtle bodies, you begin to see them. When you dream and go to those places, you can learn a lot. If you become a little bit aware, you can collect a lot of memories of your past lives and future lives, but you're not aware because you don't even know that you had a dream. Literally, your subtle body goes there. If you're unaware about it you won't be able to bring any information out of it. It's like wireless communication. Our gross body, the physical body, is the base, like a telephone. The telephone has a base in your house. Why is this human body so valuable? This base can work almost in one galaxy, it is so powerful. A computer doesn't work like that. If we send a message to the moon or to Mars, it might take a few minutes. The subtle bodies are wireless and this gross body is the base. It's called *audaric sharira*. Subtle bodies can go through the whole galaxy and it still communicates to your physical body, instantly. It's not like your subtle body is visiting somewhere beyond the stars, and it takes time to get the communication. It's instant, right away. No delay of seconds. This base is so powerful it stays connected. But all the other bases are very weak. The human body is the best base in the universe, and humans are so ignorant they don't know what they're carrying. They can go anywhere in this galaxy and stay connected. The human body is achieved after millions and millions of lives. Gaining experience and advancing slowly, through the natural evolution of the soul. All the other living beings cannot go out of their base like this. The tree is so big standing in one place its whole life, but the tree cannot go to the stars. Our subtle bodies can go anywhere.

The Ajna chakra has many sounds which activate it. Any sound which creates that kind of vibration can activate the chakra, they are not actually limited. First, you can recite "shaṁ." If you recite it you can feel it between your eyebrows; it will tickle a little bit. Recite this sound for two to three minutes. Second is "haakini." Like all the other divine sounds for the chakras, it is not a quick sound. Haaaaaaaaaaaaaaaaaaakini. The third sound is even longer, so you need to take a deep breath to make it. The sound is "aum." Inhale from your stomach, so your belly goes out all the way, and then slowly exhale all the air out as you recite: aaaaaaaaaaaaaaauuuuuuuuuuuuuuuuuuuuuuummmm. Pay attention to the sound you're making, because the "au" has to be much longer than the ending "mmmm." You don't want to quickly make the "au" and then do a very long "mmmmmm," with your lips. That is a different sound completely. For the third-eye this sound has to be very long with only a short "mmm" at the end. It is simple once you do it. It might take you five to fifteen seconds to make the sound, depending on how much air you can bring in your diaphragm.

If you recite the sound "hriṁ," with a little force as you say it, it will take you deep into your consciousness, like the *mahapranadhyana*. There is a lot to understand about mahapranadhyana. It's when you leave your body, you forget your whole body fully. You might leave for three days or five days. It's a process of how to release the subtle bodies from the physical body, and in Mahavira's time it was a popular practice. The body stays, but the subtle bodies are out. It seems like the physical body is dead, but the connection is still there. You go to the depth of consciousness and many siddhis can come to you. A siddhi is a kind of power, and most swamis are trapped into them and try to show them off, if they even have them. That is the wrong thing and has nothing to do with the path. Siddhis give the power that you can make your body change from human to animal, or big like the sky and across the stars, or small like a little bug so no one can see you. I always tell people to focus on their spirituality. Siddhis don't help you reach enlightenment, so why bother with them? That technique was related to kundalini and Parshvanath taught it. When all the chakras are awakened that is the only time you can enter into the depth of your being. In the yogic system we call it samadhi, and the very last part of samadhi is mahapranadhyana. You become totally different. You're still in the body, but you're merging with Siddha already because the knowing is the same. It's not death; you can come back from mahapranadhyana. You can come back after one day, three days, a week or a month, but the body has to be preserved in a good environment, not somewhere very hot or too cold. It has to be the right temperature. It's hard to enter into a body which is freezing, but if it's too warm then the organs and tissues and everything can start to go bad.

It was done by *Bhadrabahu*, a popular monk, and his student *Sthulibhadra*, too. Bhadrabahu was teaching this technique to Sthulibhadra, and he said not to show it to anyone. One day, Sthulibhadra's sisters, who were nuns, came to visit him. The teacher told them their brother was doing special sadhana in the forest and they could go there. Sthulibhadra knew they were coming to see him because of his siddhis, and when the sisters arrived he had turned his body into a lion. They became scared and went back to his teacher saying their brother wasn't there, only a lion. After that incident, Bhadrabahu stopped teaching. That was the end of knowledge of mahapranadhyana. Bhadrabahu wanted to teach Sthulibhadra everything, but because he began to show off to people he stopped teaching. It's not good to show you have power. It only reflects your ego. Maybe he just wanted to show his sisters what he could do, but he had promised not to show anyone. He could have just sat in meditation and they could have visited and gone back. After that, those teachings went away because no one wanted to teach it – people in that period of time wanted to show things off. They wanted to show more than do. People get a little siddhi and want to show it, like Sathya Sai Baba. He didn't even have siddhis, but was a magician and wanted to trick people into believing he had amazing powers. He was born into a magician family, I met them once. At one time south Indians belonged to the Samanic system but later on they got trapped into rituals.

Remember, the four upper chakras are ruled by God. Formless consciousness. God doesn't have a shape. It is formless like light; light is everywhere, shining everywhere. If you have that concept of God in your mind, then God is with you. It's right there waiting. Otherwise, if you are waiting to meet God on a golden chair in a paradise, then you will never meet that God. You have to open your third-eye to see it. You want to realize God? You are surrounded by God but how will you realize it? Not by talking to the mind, thinking you're talking to angels, that is just imagination and hallucination. If your body is polluted by any drugs or alcohol, nothing you experience will be the real thing. The toxins create those experiences if they're still in your body. It takes some time to clean the toxins out of your body if you are putting the effort to clean your system. Practice naturally. Clear your mind and keep your body clean. Formless consciousness is *Paramashiva*. People are mistaken that Shiva is a known person. "Parama" means "absolute," and "Shiva" means "consciousness." When your consciousness is fully awakened, or your kundalini is rising all the way up, it means your consciousness is so expanded and pure that you are closer to becoming Paramashiva – the liberated soul, formless and merged with God. Remember, your soul is formless, shapeless. It's just light. When someone becomes Siddha, it means they become Paramashiva. Siddha means you left your last body; there's no more suffering, no more karma, because the body itself is a karma. You reached enlightenment and now you are liberated from the cycle, free forever, like a bird in the sky. If you have the right concept of God in your mind, it will help you move closer.

The sense of this chakra is the sixth-sense. In English, it's called extra-sensory-perception. When this chakra is active, that kind of formless, shapeless consciousness, you begin to perceive it. How will you perceive it? You have to have the right understanding, *samayak darshan*. If you don't have right understanding of what God is, then you will never perceive it for yourself. You need the right concept first to then go beyond it. If you have the wrong concept, you will never know God.

If you can find sandalwood to cook with in your food, this will be very good for your sixth chakra. Also cook with saffron in your rice or your dishes; it affects your pituitary gland and will help it gain health.

Place lapis or sapphire over your third-eye. These stones give energy to the Ajna chakra and can balance it.

Do Shanmukhi mudra three to five times for the sixth chakra. You'll hear the sound like a low, quiet tranquil sound. Like a deep moving ocean. It will be like a deep, "aaaaaaaaauuuuuuuuuuuuuuuuuuuuuuummmm...," but not like a person is saying it. It's a very beautiful sound.

When you practice yoga to open this chakra you need to learn the baby posture, ananda balasana. Stay in this posture for five minutes and you'll be surprised the chakra begins to open. Also, you can move your eyes in clockwise circles, followed by counter-clockwise circles; this is exercising the muscles around your eyes and lower-forehead. Salamba sarvangasana, the shoulder-stand is another posture to learn. You have to be careful when practicing head-stands, shoulder-stands or any other asana that puts you in an upside-down position. Our brains have many blood vessels in them, and when all the blood is rushing into the brain in these postures it can burst the blood vessels and cause a lot of damage. I never recommend for anybody to stay in these postures for more than 1 minute maximum. 30 seconds is safer, but never more than one minute. After you come out of the posture, jump up into the air several times with your legs straight, hopping off of your toes, and throw your arms straight up to the sky; this will help the blood flow back down from your brain and you won't feel any lightheadedness or dizziness afterward. Other postures are vrkshasana, tree posture, garudasana, eagle posture, sirshasana, supported shoulder-stand, and chakrasana, wheel posture. *Jnana mudra* is a well-known mudra that will really help you to enter into your consciousness and activate your Ajna chakra. It's also known as "Gyan mudra," if you have seen it spelled this way; they are the same mudra. To create this mudra, touch the tip of your index finger to the tip of you thumb, and straighten out your other three fingers as they touch side-by-side. When you're practicing mudras, it's important to hold the mudra position for an extended period of time to feel the energy and benefit of the mudra. Don't sit for just 5 minutes with a mudra; you have to do at least 20 minutes.

The third-eye is really hit by the fragrance of lavender and rosemary. These smells open the third-eye.

The color of this chakra is indigo, so you have to find the foods which are dark blue or even some purple foods work to activate the Ajna chakra. Blueberries, eggplant, ginseng, purple potato, blackberries, shallots, boysenberries, purple grapes. There are many.

Indigo is a very good color to help the third-eye. It's a color of electricity. If you breathe in indigo with your breath, it's electric and cooling. It purifies your bloodstream. Inhale it with your breath and see that it goes all over your body, all throughout your system. Indigo controls the psychic currents of the subtle bodies. When you want to awaken spiritually and open your third-eye, visualize this color with your eyes shut. It affects another gland besides the pituitary, the pineal gland. If your vision is poor, then visualize indigo consistently and it might get better. If you have hearing or smelling problems, they can get better, too. First, visualize orange color in the ears, and then visualize indigo afterwards. This will help to heal your hearing problems. If your ears are inflamed, then instead of visualizing orange, visualize blue first. Drinking the solarized water will heal these things quickly if you can do it every day. It's helpful if you have asthma or bronchitis. It heals lung troubles, nasal disease and frequent nosebleeds. It helps pneumonia, too. If you're obsessed with people or things, indigo will help your mind calm down. With the indigo color, when your third-eye begins to open, fearlessness comes. Fearlessness means you lose the real fear, the root of it, because you begin to see the reality, the truth. The real fear disappears when the Ajna opens up. Your memory sharpens, intuition increases and you gain wisdom and vision. If the chakra is healthy you won't have many nightmares or frequent migraines and headaches, schizophrenia or anxiety, either. Sleep in the indigo light and wear purple and violet colored clothing if you need a lot of help.

Get your glass bottle, a deep dark blue – that's the closest color to indigo. Place the water in the sun all day and drink in the evening after the sun has charged it.

Work on your Ajna chakra, make it active all the time. Once your third-eye opens, these two eyes have no value anymore. You can see everything, everywhere. You are connected with the whole universe. In Sanskrit we also call the third-eye, "*bhrikuti*." "Kuti" means "cave," where shelter is. Bhrikuti is the deepest, longest cave when you go deeper and deeper into your consciousness until it opens up fully. You have to seek shelter in the path and go through the cave of consciousness. Think about this word, "bhrikuti," and close your eyes. Open your third-eye. Awaken.

SAHASRARA: THE SEVENTH CHAKRA

Chakra is the energy moving in the body. If there are blockages it means they need to cleared out, and to have knowledge of the chakra system so you're able to activate them and balance them. This way you can function well physically, emotionally and spiritually. If energy doesn't move properly it creates the feeling of discomfort, heaviness, laziness and disease.

The seventh chakra, located at the crown of your head, is called *Sahasrara*. "Sahasrara" means thousands and thousands and thousands of petals blossoming. When this chakra is open, clear, you begin to blossom. Everything in you unfolds. You expand like a lotus, multiplying thousands of petals. It is unexplainable bliss when the Sahasrara chakra is open. Unexplainable. Another name is *Brahmarandhra*. It's at the top of the head and has no element. It's only consciousness. Nearby, the highest gland in the body, is the pineal gland. It becomes very weak when the energy is not moving right in the crown of the head. It will affect your right eye; if you lose vision here, check how your chakra is. The whole upper-brain is affected. If the pineal gland is healthy, then your hair growth will be healthy as well as your nervous system. You can use these signs to check the health of your chakra.

Active Symptoms:

Enlightenment. Do you have it? This is the ultimate bliss. It never ends, it never leaves you.

Spiritual visions. Do you have any visions? They can be like seeing colors in your body, or seeing images in front of you like a movie from your past life, maybe. It can be streams of light.

Intuition. More or less everyone has it, but they don't use it or try to improve it. It's like if you're thinking of someone and then the phone rings or the door bell rings and it's them. That is real, it's not coincidence.

No prejudice. It means you don't have extreme prejudice like the Klu Klux Klan or the Nazis. Or, it can be in other ways, too, like sexism and racism.

Inactive Symptoms:

Rigid in thoughts. Are you unable or unwilling to see a different perspective? Are your beliefs engrained in you?

Unable to keep quiet. You cannot stay quiet at all.

Overactive Symptoms:

Lack concern. Either for yourself or for others, you have a lack of concern.

The sound to activate the Sahasrara is "aum," but this time you have to make the sound a different way. You inhale deeply with your stomach, let it be like a balloon, let it relax and stick out. When you begin to slowly exhale, you make the sound very long, with a deep tone, "aaaaauuuuummmmmmmmmmmmmmmmmm." The last syllable has to be the longest sound here. It is just the opposite as the sound for the Ajna chakra. This is what vibrates the crown of your skull and you can feel it, too. Place your hand on the very top of your head, and when you recite this sound you'll feel an area vibrating more than others as your mouth is closed and you're making the sound "mmmmmmmmmmmmm." That's how you can find the location of the Sahasrara chakra. You can also recite "Namo Arihantaanaṁ," to create a lot of energy. Arihanta is the enlightened person, and Arihantaanaṁ means all the enlightened people throughout the universe. All of them. So when you say, "Namo Arihantaanaṁ," you are bowing to all of the enlightened people everywhere, even if they don't live on this planet.

Remember, you are jivatma, the living being. A living being is any soul that has a body, from bacteria up to bigger bodies like elephants. They all have bodies. "Soul plus matter equals jivatma," is the formula I gave. Then, jivatma minus the matter equals paramatma, the pure soul. This is an important concept to understand. If you can understand it, you can move toward enlightenment very quickly. It will help you go further. A very old system in India, called the *Samkhya* system, talks about 24 different substances. It's a system from around 3,000 years ago, and carries some of the main principles from the Samanic tradition. If you have knowledge about these substances, you can reach enlightenment quicker, but you have to understand them very deeply. The main two substances are prakriti and *purusha*; matter and soul. There are many words for soul. In this system it is called "purusha." How do you make the soul into a pure soul, and make matter disappear? All this matter is like karma, clouds, dust, darkness, they block our light. Our soul knows a lot of things. It knows everything.

If you start to think about it you might begin to question how you can be liberated. If you don't have that concept in your mind, you won't even want to be on the spiritual path, because you don't have an understanding to imagine what the reality is. Enlightenment is unexplainable. It is a blissful state of consciousness. It's our soul's nature and it's right here with us.

This chakra is ruled by *Shivashakti*. People think that Shiva is a person and Shakti is his wife Parvathi. All the New Age followers are in illusion about it. When they meet a partner they consider themselves to be Shiva and Shakti, and they become mesmerized and fall in love. There's nothing wrong with falling in love, but it's the wrong idea to have in your head. No wonder their Sahasrara chakras are blocked. Shivashakti is when your consciousness combines with matter and pure soul. There are two substances: *jiva* is a living being, and *ajiva* is matter, it's not alive. Matter doesn't have consciousness in it; it cannot experience any sensations at all. When it merges with consciousness, only then it becomes alive. Soul is in the grip of karma. It's covered by karma. Darkness, clouds, whatever you want to call it. Somehow the soul cannot see through when it is covered by these dense clouds. The human body is the way to see through. In the Bible it says that Jesus is the only way; it's not Jesus, but the human body itself. It's a super-instrument that when combined with soul, becomes the best instrument to realize supreme consciousness – Shivashakti.

Willpower is the sense of this chakra. If you have willpower you can do anything. If you have a strong will, you can do things that other people consider impossible. You make them possible. If you have it, you can do it. It's not a sense like taste or sight. It's a special sense and it's very important to have willpower. Never read the word "impossible" as it's written. You need to read it as "I'm possible." That will take you very far in life.

Find the amethyst stone, or diamonds, and if you place them on the crown of your head for a little while it will give so much energy to the Sahasrara. They really move the energy in this chakra. Putting nutmeg in your tea or milk will also help gain the energy it needs to blossom.

For the seventh chakra you need to do Adhorechan pranayama at least 50 times, then sit and close out the outer-world. The sound of the seventh chakra is very similar to the sixth chakra's sound, but you might hear a little difference if you listen closely.

These inner-sounds will happen automatically the more you improve your kundalini, raise your intentions and balance your chakras. You have to sit quietly in calmness and peacefulness. That's the way you'll begin to listen to them. Maybe you are not familiar with the deep and tranquil stillness, so you will have to practice. It's not like you just sit and you hear them with your eyes closed. You have to be very still, your mind has to be very calm. You have to have all of your focus going deep within yourself, not being carried off by any thoughts or emotions. The sounds are an indication that will give you confidence your chakras are beginning to open.

To help this chakra through yoga, stand in vrkshasana, tree posture, for the Sahasrara to open up. Stand like a tree with your arms all the way up. It can take you higher and higher. If you want to activate all the chakras at once, learn the wheel posture, chakrasana. Children are very flexible, so it's easy for them. Anybody can do it with practice and effort. If you master this one posture and stay in it for at least three minutes, all the chakras are activated. This is the best posture for the Sahasrara chakra.

The mudra for this chakra is called the *Haakini mudra*, and it's very beneficial for your brain. To make the Haakini mudra, you simply touch all the tips of your fingers together, but no other part of the hand is touching; keep the palms and fingers apart from each other. When you touch the fingers in this way, it balances the energies on both sides of your body, and as a result, the left side of your brain which is more logical becomes equal with the right side of your brain which is more creative. It's a very good mudra to help utilize both aspects and balance them out.

Jasmine works well for aromatherapy on this chakra. Be around the smell of jasmine and your crown chakra will begin to awaken automatically.

Eat blackberries, dark blueberries, dark grapes, plums, eggplant. Some people recommend garlic, but I don't; it can create heaviness if you have too much. It's up to you, but I don't recommend to eat too much of it.

You have to visualize white color entering into your head. Sometimes you can use pink or violet, too, but they have a different meaning. Violet is for healing, pink is for compassion and love, but white is for spirituality and enlightenment. That should be your goal. Visualize a shining lotus flower with thousands of petals, so many you cannot even count them. On all the petals is the whole Sanskrit alphabet. There are 52 characters. Usually the lotus is white, but I just mentioned you have a choice of violet and pink.

White is important because it brings serenity. It's the color of purity and goodness. If you want to become pure and serene, always visualize the white color because it brings freshness and lightness. If you want to achieve bliss, work on this chakra. Its energy is like transcendence. It's called *bhavatita* – when your thoughts go away. Sometimes yogis close their ears with their thumbs so the outer-world cannot be heard at all, and

Muslim people sometimes pray like this. They got it from the yogic system. They used to see the yogis doing this a long time ago when they were in that area. Most of the eastern religions carry many techniques from the yogic and Samanic system. What happens when you can't hear the outer sounds? You are fully quiet, and you might begin to hear the inner sounds. Quiet, long humming: mmmmmmmmmmmmmmmm. It's very soothing and beautiful. When you begin to hear this sound it means the top of your head is becoming clear. Bring all the white light into your head, visualize it there. See all the peace and stillness coming into you. You begin to have wisdom, inspiration and awareness when this chakra is open. It comes automatically, because white light heals mental sicknesses and clears confusions and doubts. You have to be clear of confusion to know who you are. Wear white clothes. In China, white is the color of mourning. It's the best time to get enlightened when someone you know dies, because you begin to think about your life and that you will die soon, too. You have the opportunity to go so deep through all of your pain that you come out on the other side of it. It's fully gone then. White represents enlightenment. One day you might get it.

If you really want enlightenment, there is a secret you have to understand about the Sahasrara chakra. There are four kinds of people who will never reach enlightenment, because they are suffocating their chakra. In Western culture, the oldest religion is Judaism, and somehow they have yogic teachings in their traditions. Many religions were formed after yoga so they have a lot of the teachings, but they became distorted over time. In Judaism they wear a little *yarmulke* (yamaka) on their head always. It sits on the crown chakra, and "yamaka" in Sanskrit means "messenger of Death." It symbolizes that before your message of death comes to you, you have to open this chakra. They started wearing it like that and never stopped. It is suffocating their Sahasrara chakra so much and they don't even know what is happening to them. It's supposed to be a reminder to work on the seventh chakra and let spirituality unfold, but they forgot it. They carry the tradition still, but no longer carry the meaning.

The second group who are never going to be enlightened and reach God are the bishops, the pope, the cardinals and others like them. Unless you need protection from the harsh sun or other weather, that's a different thing, but don't cover your head all the time with big caps and hats. Enlightenment means there is no difference between God and that person who is enlightened. It's just a matter of time before their body dies and they become liberated and merge with God. It was a teaching but they forgot it. All these people are keeping themselves in the dark because they won't let their chakras open. In Arab countries they wear turbans in the name of religion. It's okay if they wear it outside because of the environment they live in, but they wear it all the time, and in the name of God. They say they want to be with God, but they just block themselves instead. When you get to your home at least take your turban off, or whatever you may be wearing, so air can move around your head.

The fourth group is all the Sikhs. They will never reach enlightenment because they suffocate it doubly. Their books seem very good, and they seem like they are good people, but they are suffocating their crown chakra. According to their religion, they don't cut their hair, and when they go out they wrap it around the top of their head. And on top of that they wrap a turban around it. It's their religion, but they don't know what is happening to them. The same goes for Kundalini Yoga practitioners. It doesn't make sense that they want to activate their kundalini, yet they are blocking their seventh chakra. Only wear those things for protection from weather or if you require it at work. That doesn't do any harm. But in the name of religion or yoga, never keep your head covered all the time like this. It will be very difficult for all the thousands of petals in you to blossom.

There is another secret which Parshvanath was teaching. It can bring the bliss of God quickly and you will taste it. Learn how to do the *Kechari mudra*. It's difficult to learn, but you twist your tongue so the tip reaches in your palate at the back of your mouth. It's near the nasal passage. If you can hold it here and press your tongue in, eventually all the nectar will come to you. You will really taste it. Parshvanath taught it and it was collected in the yogic system. All his teachings were lost but I am bringing them to light again. This technique comes from him. You'll be surprised how quick you enter into meditation if you practice this and master it the correct way.

CHAKRAS FOR BUSINESS

Now that you know how to balance your chakras safely, it is important to learn how they can help you in life. Chakras can play an important role in improving or developing businesses. If your chakras are not working, you might not be successful. You have to understand that they need to be balanced. The most perfect business people who have a lot of success have an open heart chakra. If it's closed, the business doesn't work. I will tell you, you cannot be in a business being like a rock. You have to be soft. If you're like a rock or stone, it means it's not going to work. Your energy will be totally distracted and no one will pay attention to you. When your chakras are aligned, you're not like a rock. You're more soft. If your chakras are aligned you'll be smiling. When you smile, people are interested in you. If you're not open-hearted, then you cannot converse with other people. It will be difficult for you in your business.

Japanese are very successful in business. They forward bend (bow) three times, and people don't get it. Why do they do it? The heart chakra has to be open before you can bend. If your heart is not open you can't do it. Forward bending shows the person is humble, and you might want to talk to him or her. When you meet someone, if you don't introduce somehow, like, hi, hello, or whatever your system is, if you don't do it or shake hands, then the person might have a bad impression of you to begin with. All things have to be soft. Soft touch. If your chakras are not aligned you're very depressed. Even if you go to meet someone to work with their company or partnership, your eyes are dull, you sound not interested. Eye contact is very important. Soften the whole body, don't be like a rock. If somebody is talking to you, you nod or do some kind of body gesture to show you're listening. Everyone wants to be heard and acknowledged.

For business purposes, the black color is a powerful color. It's not bad. Where all colors meet, it's black. We need black. It can be dark like navy blue, too. Dark colors absorb everything. Use the green color to open your heart. You cannot be soft unless your heart is open. Your heart has to be fully open. If you have money and are a lady, put on the pendant of a real emerald, it will attract other people and improve business. It has to touch over your heart center. It has to be a big piece, not very small. Your chakra will be balanced with this. If you're a man you can wear a ring. A gold ring with an emerald. It will attract business because the green energy opens your heart and softens you. You're no longer like a rock; you'll smile, you'll be open-hearted. You will bend forward, your touch will be very soothing and peaceful. You will talk to the person with good eye contact.

If we don't listen we lose a lot of things. We miss a lot of things. Listening is important. By listening you can be very knowledgeable. If a person is not starting a business conversation right away, then talk about traveling, movies, gardening, or something else. If you're not interested in listening, you cannot improve your business. You won't be interested unless your heart is open. Shine your heart chakra. Here are sounds to recite: "Namo Uvajjhaayaanam." This sound will create tremendous green light in you. You become a soft person. If a boss is very hard like a rock, no one will like them. A boss has to be hard, but only sometimes; he or she has to be soft and friendly to

communicate and relate to people, too. If you want success in your business, open your heart.

First concentrate on your fourth chakra, then the first chakra. The first chakra is red. If you are a business woman, wear a red skirt or shirt sometimes. This goes for the businessmen, too. If you can't wear a red shirt, wear a red tie. That red will help open and balance your first chakra. Then you concentrate on the third – Manipura, the navel center of the body. That has to be very open and bright yellow. If you have anything bright yellow, or orangish yellow, wear that. In the winter, wear an orange or yellow scarf. Anything yellow, it will help to open your chakra. While working on the second chakra, Svadhisthana, try to wear orange clothing if you can. Even a little bit of orange on a tie, or scarf, or other garments. Fifth is expression and is light blue. Anything light blue on your body, it will help open your chakra and balance it. Seventh chakra is white. Wear a white shirt, or anything else white. You already have some dark.

How to attract the business? Follow what I mentioned about these chakras. Go in this order: Anaahat (heart chakra), Muladhara (root chakra), Manipura (navel chakra), Svadhisthana (sacral chakra), Vishuddhi (throat chakra), Sahasrara (crown chakra), and Ajna (wisdom chakra). Heart is green. Root is red. Navel is yellow. Sacral is orange. Throat is light blue. Crown is white, and the third-eye is indigo. If you follow this way of alignment you'll be surprised. Remember the sound "Namo Uvajjhaayanam," and recite it 108 times, daily. The combination of these sounds creates automatically green light in you and your heart will be open. You'll already have a smile on your face, a beautiful touch and good eye contact. It makes other people interested in you. When you start conversing with people don't just talk about your own family, people don't like it. It's better to talk about different things, like these days, if a person is very healthy talk about fitness or yoga, try to see what the person likes. If they look intellectual maybe talk about science or educational things, learning. Keep your chakras always active. The chakras will work for you and bring business to you when you are aligned properly and balanced, because your whole system will be clear and working much better.

CHAKRAS FOR RELATIONSHIPS

Relationships are important in human lives. If you fail in relationships, you fail in society. Even though you will keep talking about your good relationship with God, you will not be good in society. Let me tell you a story. There was a man once, and he was always looking at the stars; it was his passion. He was always looking to try and find a new planet in the sky. One night, he was walking along and looking up into the twinkling stars and he walked right into an elderly lady who was walking.

"What are you doing here?" she asked him.

"Hey, can't you see that I'm searching for planets? You're in my way."

She was a very wise lady and she said to him, "Can I tell you one thing? First learn to walk on the Earth, then you go look for other planets."

You have to also live in reality and not be lost in your own world, in your imagination and things that you enjoy. If you don't know how to make successful relationships, you will be broken-hearted all the time, with your family, friends, or other people.

Relationships don't work unless your first chakra is open. The Muladhara chakra is red. In your blood there has to be a lot of red blood cells. It means you have good blood circulation. When the body is active, then you begin to feel for someone. If your body is lazy, you don't feel like doing anything, just lying down, even though you feel lonely, eat a lot and get depressed. You're not grounded or balanced at all. Relationships don't start in the heart like people think. You need to be very active first. You need the energy to be involved in life. Otherwise you won't feel good about yourself or anyone else. You can become jealous, hateful, and resentful.

Wear red colors, and it will help create that energy in you. If you're a lady, get a red ruby pendant, or a red shirt or skirt. You have to be very physically active. Relationships won't improve without healthy energy in your root chakra.

Repeat the divine sound, "daakini," all the time. The more you do it, the more it opens. You begin to feel for other people, and you feel grounded at the same time. This chakra has to be very strong. You will have a lot of energy, and you can move further. Visualize red inside of you, filling your body. Live with nature and be in nature a lot. Your body and mind will become very active and clear.

Next work on your fourth chakra, the heart chakra. When the fourth chakra begins to open, love, excitement, and all emotions will come to the surface. When there is love and excitement you begin to feel alive. Fifth chakra is next, the throat chakra. Suddenly, you begin to be like a poet, even if you don't consider yourself a poet, the way you speak will be very expressive and beautiful. Next work on the second chakra and wear orange colors a lot. It will help you share your thoughts and emotions. The Manipura, the third chakra, needs to be balanced following the second chakra. Its color is yellow. How will you express words if you will wait forever? If your heart is open and you feel love for someone, but you never express it, how do you know it will work or not? Maybe you two are close friends for 10 years, but you never expressed it, so they don't know how much you feel for them. You need to open your self-expression. Then the sixth chakra. Practice tratka, the ancient technique from the Samanic system. Once your sixth chakra is improved, the energy in your crown chakra begins to expand. That energy will attract the person you're looking for.

That is the way you can improve your relationships through your chakras. Communication is key to relationships. Through balanced chakras, you will learn how to express yourself. You will be able to talk about goals, things you like, what you do, all of these things in your life will come out easily. Always smile. The energy from the first chakra radiates through all the chakras, and that's how the relationship forms.

CHARAS FOR EDUCATION

We need higher-education. When you are educated, you develop your mind more and can gain a new world-view perspective. Education helps you to think and ask questions. For higher education you need to align all of your chakras. First start by opening up your third-eye this way you are able to concentrate and absorb everything that you learn. This chakra, the Ajna chakra, has to be very strong.

If you are in school now, you require a lot of energy and focus in order to take in everything that you are learning. Not only take in, but apply as well. Unfortunately, students experience a lot of stress and distractions. They might be distracted because of friends, work, family and other responsibilites. You need to have peace within you and balance among your friends, family, work and responsibilities to have a clear mind. When your mind is clear, there is space for you to learn. A lot of stress comes from the family.

What does family mean? Father, And, Mother, I, Love, You. That is your family. If you say to your father and mother, "I love you," as an adult they will be very happy with you. When you're happy, they're happy. When they are happy, you are happy. Do your best to keep peace with your family, and a lot of stress will be reduced; if you're raised in a good family environment, you'll be able to keep a lot of focus on yourself.

To increase concentration and intellect, focus on your third-eye. Use the indigo color; it has to be strong in you. Visualize, breathe in and swallow the indigo color into you. It will make your third-eye stronger, and when it's strong you will begin to see better results in focus, clarity, concentration, and reduced stress. To increase concentration practice the tratka technique. Or, another technique, where you focus on the candle flame in a very dark room to become an expert in visualization. It will help you so much.

After working on the sixth chakra, work on your third chakra. At night, if you have a diamond, place the diamond on your navel. It will increase your stamina so that you can focus on your studies for even 12 hours continuous without getting tired. But without the third chakra being balanced, it will be difficult to sit still. Practice any of the techniques in the chakra system; you don't need to use a diamond. After working on the third chakra, focus on the second chakra. You will be and feel more stable, and less restless. Then work on the fifth chakra. You will express what you're learning or thinking very well. Creativity will happen, too. If you need to give a presentation, focus on your fifth chakra in advance in order to build the color there. Then work on the seventh chakra next. Do some kind of sarvangasana, shoulder-stand, for no more than one minute, then stand up again and jump in the air seven times to let the blood come down from your brain. As you jump to the air, throw your arms straight up above your head, all the way stretched out. Blood goes to your brain and it's not healthy to practice certain yoga postures which take you upside down, for more than a minute. After the seventh, work on your heart chakra. Your heart has to be last to work on in the case of education. If you're in college or high school and your heart is too open, you'll find love everywhere, get distracted and not complete your education. It's important to work on it last. If you're a girl and have blue sapphire or blue topaz necklace, it will help you a lot. If you are a boy, you can wear a blue shirt or blue stone in a ring. Touch the blue stone at night to your forehead. Your focus will increase tremendously. Work on your chakras in this order for help in education: Ajna, Manipura, Svadhisthana, Vishuddhi, Sahasrara, Anaahat, Muladhara. For education the first chakra is not as important, although it's important for your life. When you're young, your first chakra is generally always active, so you just need to balance and maintain it. Work on the chakras in this given order and your studies and education will be positively affected.

INDIVIDUALITY OF SOUL

When you dissolve all the karma, you are free. If your energy is moving the right way and you can keep your chakras balanced, then you will flow in positivity and go closer to the spiritual path. That is the way to burn your karmas. You have to understand and go deep inside to find out who you really are and what this life is about. That's why in the Jain system they say, "Appa so paramappa." "Appa" means the "soul," and "paramappa" means "God." Soul is God. And everyone is telling that. Even if you ask a Christian, they will tell you they are children of God. What does that mean? Appa so paramappa: children of God. They are saying the same truth, but in a different way. The only difference is they don't go any deeper into it. They don't have that kind of thinking. If they begin to think deeper and deeper, then they will follow the real *sayam*, discipline. They will follow the real path. Otherwise, they will just keep repeating that they are children of God. That's it. In the *Upanishadas*, they have the statement, "*Aham Brahmasmi,*" "I am God." Mahavira said, "Appa so paramappa." It is a very shaking, controversial and revolutionary statement to say, "I am God." Maybe Mahavira's statement is not as strong, but they are both true. Remember, it is not like "I am God," with an ego. If the ego is there, that person is in illusion. When someone is not on the spiritual path, they are just atma, just soul. But when that person is on the path and they take diksha, they get initiated into monkhood, then that soul becomes mahatma, a great soul. When the great soul follows the path and goes through their own experiences, improves themselves and dissolves their karma, what is going to happen? Then they become paramatma. "Param" means "absolute." Now there is nothing left to blossom. The soul is fully blossomed, like a beautiful flower, and there is nothing left to blossom. The soul's journey becomes great, then the greatest, but you have to go through it with effort. We usually call it "paramatma," not "God." They share the same meaning.

All the liberated souls create God. When a soul is liberated and merged with God, they remain individual still. If you go through the Jain teachings, the real teachings, you will be surprised. They are so democratic, up to the end. Even when you become Siddha, when you merge with God, your light still remains separate. Otherwise what will you enjoy if you dissolve into God? Suppose you become a part of a tree. A tree is God, suppose, and you become one leaf on that tree, what will you enjoy? You become a little tiny thing, a part of the whole thing. Your individuality is taken away. It means God is a dictator. When God is a dictator, that God is not God at all.

If you will read the Jain system thoroughly, deeply, you will see that even when you merge with God your individuality will be there forever. It is a light, like in your room, suppose. How does it work? There's one candle, two candles, hundreds of candles, thousands of candles, and light merges with the light. But there is a way now to see where the light is the individual light. You can make it separate these days. There was no way in the old days to make it separate. Now, by computers, we have technology and we can see where one candle's particles of light are. They are reflecting the particles – that is light. Otherwise we cannot see the light. Light is not visible. People's dilemma is that they think light is visible. Light only shows others whatever is there. What is the light? You cannot see light itself. We are seeing what is reflected, all the particles of matter are reflected by this light. You can see your computer, or your desk, or a book; it is just a reflection. If there's no light then it doesn't get reflected and we cannot see what it is. So, what the light does is reflect the particles of matter. One candle is reflecting, and another hundred candles are reflecting at the same time, but we can find the light from individual candles these days. In the same way, the soul remains independent even when it merges with God, with all the other liberated souls. So, your individuality never disappears. Your democracy is never taken away. If you go to the Hindu systems, you are gone. Because they say when you merge with God, that's it, you disappear. They say that one drop merges with the ocean and you become the ocean. In the Jain system they say that all the drops remain independent, but they create the ocean together. What makes the ocean? All the tiny drops of water. If you take every little drop of water away from the ocean, the ocean is gone fully. Who makes God? Siddhas make God. The liberated souls. If there are no Siddhas, then there is no God. Siddhas are like the drops of water, and they create a big ocean called God, what we call paramatma.

Sometimes I tell people that God is in everything. Because it is made of all souls who are blossomed, who are fully flowered already. God is everything. There is nothing left in this world which is not God. And I ask people sometimes, what do they eat. You eat divinity. What do you hear? You hear divinity. If you have vision, the real vision, then you can see the divinity, otherwise maybe some things look ugly to you. The person who becomes a saint thinks the world is very beautiful. They say, "All the stars, the Milky Way, moons and suns and trees, the oceans and mountains, wow. It is so beautiful." Another person says, "This mountain is just a pile of rocks. It's so hard. Why? There is no softness in it." They can find things depending on how they look at them. The world can be very beautiful, or it can be very ugly. But with the real vision, you see past it. So, if you merge with God, why are you putting the efforts if you will not be individual at all? What is the meaning of it? The Hindu idea of God is like that; they will send you back again. You never get salvation. You never become liberated. Forget about it. It's not in your hands. If you read in the Bhagavad Gita, what Hindus believe is the holiest book, nothing is in your hands. In God's hands everything goes. They live by "God's grace" or "God's will." God's hands will bring you here to this life, then call you there, then send you back again. It means whatever efforts you're putting are useless. If you're a Hindu and you don't know any other system, you will be roaming in the dark forever. I don't blame those swamis that they don't reach enlightenment. Why? Because they don't have the idea to achieve it in the first place. They don't think that way. They have just the idea to become a saint, a pure son of God, that's it. And if God calls you, God can send you back again. It means God is everything and you are nothing, so what do your efforts mean? Nothing. They are useless. When you are nothing what is the meaning of putting any effort? Always remember, that boss who keeps their employees as employees is not a boss. A real boss will make his or her employees the boss one day, a partner. That is a good boss. A swami is supposed to make a person a swami, not keep them as a slave like their God does. How will they do it if they are not a real swami to start with? You will always be like a slave.

You merge with God, you get thrown away again. Then you'll suffer again. That's the wrong idea. We are carrying a very wrong idea amongst today's cultures, but many religions carry it everywhere. India is one of those places. It's better to find the truth, and it's nowhere. You have to blossom yourself. How do you keep blossoming yourself? You have to put efforts, and remember, even if you merge with God, you remain independent still. God has such a big heart that your freedom cannot be taken away. Never. That's why it's God. If God takes your freedom away, then what is the meaning of God? The guru is a real guru who makes their disciple a guru one day. God is the same. So, the training of the disciple is to take them higher to become enlightened. That is the meaning of guru; spread the lights everywhere. God is the same thing. It's not like what Hindus say, "It's God's will." Then, if God gets bored, God will throw you away again into the world. It means you will never become liberated.

Why do all these Hindus always go to die on the bank of the Ganges River? Hundreds and thousands of them. I've met many people there. When I ask why they are sitting there, they reply, "Because we're waiting to die. If we die on the bank of the river we achieve moksha." I always tell them, if that's the case, what about all those fish, frogs and turtles? They live in the river and die in the river, so they are already better than you.

Wake up. People don't want to hear the truth. They still keep teaching those things. There is no easy way. Until you go through the death, you don't know what death is. Until you die, you don't know what dying is. Until you suffer, you don't know what suffering is. Unless you die before you die, you don't get moksha, liberation. You have to die the real death, not like sitting on the bank of a river. The Mississippi River is even longer than the Ganges and they are crazy about it in India. In some aspects it's good water because near the Himalayas it touches many plants and becomes like a medicine, but not if you go to Varanasi – it's already polluted there, and millions of people are crazy to dip in that water. The truth is very difficult to hear, difficult to digest it and difficult to follow. It's not just that you know the truth. No. It is very difficult to digest. How will you know it if you can't even hear it? Swamis will put these three big stripes across their foreheads and make a big fire and all the Hindus think that is a good Baba. At night what do they do? They smoke marijuana and use drugs. All night long, because if they are sitting in the cold weather, totally naked, they will die otherwise. They don't know the path, they just depend on Krishna only. Krishna hasn't even liberated himself, yet. All Hindus and Jains believe Krishna will come back once again.

Many people are ignorant. How many people carry the real path even in India? Ideas are very good there, but how many among them follow the real path? They enjoy hearing that Guru Nanak said this, or the Gita said this or some other person or book said this. Yes, they might have said it, but are you following it? Sikhs hear, "*Hai Bhee Sach, Aadi Sach...*" over and over. They just hear it again and again. They cannot even pronounce it the right way and they sing it over and over. Maybe they're not even reading the right words, because they say always "*Jugaadi Sach,*" but there is no such a word. It is "*Yugaadi Sach.*" "Ya" became "Ja." It is not even "Sach," it is "*Sathya.*" "Sach" means "Sathya" – *Adi Sathya, Yugaadi Sathya.* That is the original pronunciation, but they go around singing it all the time – incorrectly – and don't even know about it. It was so simple but they distorted the words. They say: *Adi Sach,* God is the first; *Jugaadi Sach,* God is since the beginning; *Hai Bhee Sach,* God is Truth; *Nanak Ho Si Bhee Sach,* God will remain true always. That's the meaning they put, but it was not the original. It was totally different before. It was: *Aadi Sathya,* Adinath (first Tirthankara) was true; *Yugaadi Sathya,* he was the beginning of this era – "Yuga" means "era." *Hai Bhee Sathya,* he is true because he was enlightened. Tirthankara Adinath is still true and his teachings are still available. And in the future, Nanak was telling them, he will remain true. That is the real meaning but not a single Sikh knows it, because they cannot understand Sanskrit.

Anytime you are learning about spirituality, it is best to go deep into it and try to understand it and grasp the meaning fully. If there's an enlightened master available, then don't wait to visit them. They can give you the right guidance for your individual path, for your own soul. Soul is never-ending; it cannot be put out like the light from a candle, the light from the sun, or the light from a bulb. It shines forever, and you have to make your goal to realize this light; what is it? Where is it coming from? That is the path you need to be on. Don't waste any more of your time stuck in *pramada*. Pramada is all of your negative thoughts, all of your hate and frustration, your anger, sadness, pride and ego, jealousy, greed, and so on. You don't need to be in these any longer. It's time for you to be on the path and awaken your soul.

PART IV:
WHAT'S NEXT?

CREATING YOUR PRACTICE

Spirituality is practicality. Remember that. You have learned a lot in this book, but all learning needs to be applied in order to see results. Many times I come across intellectual people that have read a lot of book, lots of scriptures, and are well-versed in various schools of thought. If you look at them and how they live their life, you can see that they know many things and have collected a lot of knowledge, but they might lead a miserable and unhappy life. Why? Because they didn't practice.

I want you to grow. I want you to advance. My wish for you is to reach enlightenment and moksha. That is why I have dedicated time to put this book together for you. When I see potential, I put efforts. I know that you can be benefited by knowing and deeply understanding all that I have shared with you. To be benefited, you must put efforts. The guru-student relationship is two ways. Guru puts efforts into the student by sharing their knowledge. Students put efforts into the spiritual path by practicing what they have been taught. Both guru and student are happy, because now there is one more soul in this world that is on the path and can help light the path for others.

First thing, before you begin your practices, read this book in full one more time. It may seem like a lot to you, but let a week pass then read through again. I say this, because you were in one mood when you first read the book, and the second time you will be in a different state and will pick up on more things. Once you have read the book at least twice, then proceed to practice the techniques I have shared with to work on your chakras.

Many people get confused on where to start with the chakras. Do you work from the first chakra up? Should you work on one chakra per week or per month? I will say it is up to you. However, here are some things to remember.

First, start with the chakra that seems the weakest to you. If they all seem weak equally, then I would suggest starting with balancing out the first chakra. By now you know that if there is no energy in the first chakra, there won't be much flow of energy to rise from downward to upward. It requires a lot of energy and force. If you do know your weakest chakra, write them down in order of priority from weakest to strongest and work on your chakras in that order.

Second, make the commitment to work on your chakras for at least 41 days. After 21 days, you will begin to see some results of your efforts, depending how much time and effort you've put in. Remember, what you put in, you get out. It will be a very big milestone for you to complete the 41 days of chakra practice.

Third, just because you work on your chakras one time doesn't mean they will stay balanced forever. Like all things on the path, you must continue to put efforts in raising your energy, understanding the teachings more, and deepening your meditation. You should check in on your chakras at least once to twice a month to see what state they are in. If you notice they are imbalanced, work on them.

Fourth, have patience with yourself. Do your practices whole-heartedly; if you practice with expectation and force, the results will be totally different. Keep your path simple. Don't get stuck into achieving enlightenment and liberation right away. Step by step you will reach your goal. If you make huge leaps, you will fall. I don't want that for you. Slow and steady wins the race.

Fifth, if you want personal guidance from me, for your spiritual path, your chakras, and to awaken your soul, meet me at Siddhayatan near Dallas, Texas. Sign up for a retreat so that I can guide you personally. I don't know how many times I have helped people because their energy went the wrong way and went crazy after practicing chakra techniques given by "experts, masters and gurus." If this seems like you, I can help you become balanced and connect you to yourself again.

If you are feeling overwhelmed after reading all these teachings and practices twice, I am providing you a sample sadhana (spiritual practice) schedule for you to follow. If you don't have as much time or your health doesn't permit it, then adjust it. Be flexible, but be consistent.

A 30-minute practice

Before sunrise:

- Deep breathing outside visualizing the chakra's color that you are working on.
- Practice your breathing techniques.
- Practice yoga.
- Practice mantra and divine sounds.
- Meditate for 10 minutes on the chakra color.
- Fill your chakra color bottle with water and place outside where there won't be any shade.

Before sunset:

- Drink solarized water.

A 20-minute practice

Before sunrise:

- Deep breathing
- Practice your breathing techniques.
- Practice mantra and divine sounds.
- Fill your chakra color bottle with water and place outside where there won't be any shade.

Before sunset:

- Drink solarized water

Evening:

- Meditate 5 minutes on the chakra color.

A 10-minute practice

Morning:

- Breathing techniques
- Practice mantra and divine sounds
- Fill your chakra color bottle with water and place outside where there won't be any shade.

Before sunset:

- Drink solarized water

Evening:

- Meditate 5 minutes on the chakra color.

A 5-minute practice

Anytime:

- Breathing techniques
- Practice mantra and divine sounds
- Fill your chakra color bottle with water and place outside

where there won't be any shade.

You may have noticed that the common practices are daily breathing (for your own health and health of chakra), mantra and divine activation sounds, and drinking the solarized water. It is up to you how you would like to create your schedule. I highly suggest creating a 41-day calendar on the computer, print it out to hang on the wall, or create notification reminders on your cell phone, this way you do it every day. Every day you practice, cross out the day, this will help you stay on track, keep you motivated in any case you become lazy, and inspire you to complete your 41 days. Never give up. Doing something is better than doing nothing at all.

Before starting your practices, I have one request for you. Take the first step to be truly spiritual. Be vegetarian.

IMPORTANCE OF VEGETARIANISM

I always suggest that becoming a vegetarian is the very first step if you want to move towards spirituality. This is the message I want to give to you. Why? Because you begin to gain respect for all living beings, and when you feel respect for even a little spider or a fly, how will you continue to eat meat when you understand that all of these animals feel pain? Animals that are more developed have all the five senses, plus a mind. When somebody kills them, it's like torture for them and they don't understand why their life is being taken away. They have very bad feelings and their whole system changes when they're killed. It's a different story when they die naturally. When they're killed, their whole system is shaken up and it creates a lot of harmful things in their flesh and blood. Adrenaline and fear is pumped into their blood. Whoever eats that animal gets all of these toxins into their body and even just one time it creates so much pollution. It damages the human body. People become very heavy-minded, thinking the wrong way which doesn't help them, and they feel like their body is not comfortable for them. And those people who are trying to do meditation and spiritual practices, they think they can reach enlightenment without being a vegetarian, they are fully wrong.

How do they expect to reach the highest state of consciousness and awaken their soul when they cannot even respect other living beings? The soul never wakes up in that kind of body which is damaged with toxins; it's not possible because that body is very weak. The spiritual path requires tremendous energy.

These animals with five senses and a mind feel a lot of things; not just physical pain, but they have the ability to think a little bit, too. They become confused, anxious, very fearful and terrified. They know what is about to happen to them.

Then there are living beings that are less developed, with just four senses. They can't hear, but have eyes, a nose, a mouth and they have the sense of touch as well. They still can feel a lot of pain. Never eat these things either. In Thailand and China, many Asian countries, they're eating a lot of these four-sensed living beings. These are like scorpions and spiders.

There are three-sensed, two-sensed and one-sensed living beings. One-sensed living beings are still alive but they are in an unconscious state. It means they feel a little pain, but because they're unconscious it doesn't affect them, and they don't know what is happening. This state is totally different from a five-sensed living being. Like a tree; a tree has one sense, to feel, but it doesn't know what is going on, if someone is cutting a branch or running their fingers along it's bark or climbing on them, it has no idea. When a person has a problem and needs to have an operation, the doctor will give them anesthesia. After that, when they're unconscious, the doctor can cut their bones and they won't even feel any pain. It's like that. So, the one-sensed living beings are the lowest category of living beings. They don't feel any pain, and they don't suffer.

Soul lives in the body. Humans have five senses and the most developed mind, so we can go deep into something and try to understand

it. We can think about our suffering and try to find out where it comes from, and if you don't want it anymore, you can make that decision to go through it and end it. This is in our hands if we want it. To awaken the soul, we have to be living in the human body, and we have to feed this body. You have to choose the category of food which doesn't feel any pain, and take only what you need. If you want one apple, take one apple, don't cut the whole tree. If you want one vegetable, take one. This way you don't destroy the whole thing. These days, the way that commercial slaughterhouses operate, a single hamburger patty can contain meat from hundreds and even thousands of cows, as all of the meat is mixed together in the machines that are used. How many living, breathing animals suffered as they were killed for your little burger? If you had to kill all of those cows with your own hands for a hamburger patty, would you do it? When somebody wants just a small piece of chicken, they have to kill it; they can't just take the piece they want, like a plant. A chicken has five senses. It is torture for that chicken when a person wants to eat it. The people who eat lobsters are even worse. The lobsters are put in a pot of boiling water. That is torture and they feel so much pain there. Imagine someone picking you up and dropping you in boiling water; your whole body will cook from the inside out. Those lobsters have to go through that kind of pain when somebody wants to eat one.

If someone wants to really be on the spiritual path, the first thing they have to think is to start eating the food which is the lowest level of consciousness, and doesn't feel the pain of what is happening to them. I strongly suggest people to become vegetarian. How can you consider yourself spiritual otherwise?

The second reason I want to share with you is when you eat fruits, vegetables and grains, which are considered the lightest food, they are digested very easily in your body. On the other hand, meat takes three days to digest because our intestines are very long. It sits in your body for three entire days (even longer if you eat a lot of meat), and it creates a lot of trouble for you. This is how people get many diseases. Imagine those who have meat as part of their 3 meals per day? The body doesn't get rest, the energy is stuck, and they are susceptible to health problems. Whatever light food you eat, it passes through the body usually in a maximum of 12 hours. If you pick the lightest foods to eat, maybe only 6 hours and it's completely through your system. Your body becomes light and healthy. A light body creates a light mind which can take you into meditation. The mind will cooperate with you and you become more balanced; you don't have to do so much battling with your thoughts. You can go deep into samadhi, but the first condition is that you try to respect living beings which are more developed. You have to respect all living beings, but you need to eat something in order to survive. Find those things which are the lowest level of consciousness.

People who think meat is good for the brain are wrong. More than 90% of Hindu and Jain Indians are vegetarian and they are very intelligent. Even in America, 43% of doctors are Indian, and many of them are vegetarian. There is a wrong concept that meat is necessary for the human body. Albert Einstein, he was considered a genius on the planet, and he was a vegetarian. Also, many people consider Mahatma Gandhi a great person, and he was also vegetarian. You have to adopt vegetarianism and your mind will be light, your body will be light and you will feel light and flowing always. You need to learn to make light food, sattvic food. Vegetarian people can become divine if they have the right spiritual guidance at the same time. They can become like that, because they're already moving towards the path by having respect for living beings. Not to harm anything, that should be your idea; just have what you need for survival. The food is coming from the soil, so you are in contact with the earth already. And when you are an earthly person, it means you respect your mother, because the earth is the mother and she nurtures us and provides everything that we need to thrive. If you want to be spiritual, the first step is to be vegetarian. It will make you peaceful and divine, and bring something unique into your consciousness, because you begin to see clearly and think in the right direction. Remember, soul can only awaken in the body which is pure and free of toxins.

As a vegetarian, your body will be healthier and purified. You will be practicing nonviolence. Working on your chakras alone is helpful to an extent, but without being vegetarian, your energy will be heavy, stuck and not flow upwards towards your goal. Your goal is to awaken, shine and become enlightened. Vegetarianism is a requirement for such a path.

FINAL THOUGHTS

One day, my Chief Disciple, Sadhvi Siddhali Shree asked me a wise question. She asked, "If you went into silence in this moment for the rest of your life, what would be your last words or teachings?"

I answered, "Siddha."

Siddha means "liberated soul." The goal of your spiritual path is to be liberated. That is why I share these teachings and experiences with you, because I want you to become liberated one day. Why continue living in the cycle of birth and death, to only suffer and remain in illusion? The purpose of your life is to awaken, to get on the real path, and after time and effort become liberated.

To be on the real path, you must first begin to dissolve and let go of the beliefs and ideologies that prevent you from growing and getting on the right track. Currently, there are so many misleading teachings and teachers out there that are harmful to your path and will keep you in the dark. They are in the dark themselves, but it won't appear that way. That is why it was important to share in detail with you the history of spirituality this way you know and understand the truth — how the path started, how it got distorted and how to be on the real one.

Since this book is about chakra awakening it was important to share with you the lost teachings and techniques of the first kundalini master, 23rd Tirthankara Parshvanath. The main teachings of the Tirthankaras are to help you become liberated. It is difficult to achieve enlightenment and liberation if you are practicing the wrong things. Parshvanath shared the leshya system (chakra system) for spiritual practitioners at that time because they were interested in new spiritual tools to help them advance. He taught by having the purest intentions, you create a lot of positive colors in your aura, uplift your energy, deepen your understanding, become healthier, and increase your awareness – all of which are important to realize your soul. By living in lower thinking with negative intentions, not only does it create violence in and around you, but it also prevents you from growing.

Practicing chakra awakening techniques without a solid spiritual foundation is like skydiving without a parachute. It doesn't make sense. Before practicing any techniques, you need a solid understanding of spirituality so that you can lead and live a spiritual life, slowly and steadily moving towards awakening, enlightenment and liberation.

Working on the chakras alone does not take you to enlightenment and liberation. It is the spiritual and soul understanding that does. The chakra system is merely a tool that when combined with true spiritual understanding can help you achieve the highest states of consciousness. There are other tools to help you achieve enlightenment and liberation; however, tools by themselves take you nowhere. Tools without understanding are powerless.

If you are a dedicated truth seeker and are focused on liberating yourself, my advice to you is to first be a non-violent person. By becoming non-violent your intentions, thoughts, actions and speech are pure. When you live a pure life, there is no way for you to collect karma and pollute your soul. Another requirement for enlightenment and liberation is being vegetarian. Don't let the myths and misconceptions of vegetarianism fool you, like needing protein from animals in order to be healthy. Eating meat and eggs doesn't liberate your soul. If you are serious about your spiritual path, you will become vegetarian. Through nonviolence all aspects of your life will begin to shift and transform in a positive way. When living a non-violent life, you are balanced, calm, fearless, and peaceful.

By being non-violent, practicing spirituality whole-heartedly, and working on your chakras, not only will you change yourself, but you will change the world.

Liberate yourself.

Become Siddha.

YOGA ASANAS

Yoga postures, *asanas*, are very important for chakra and kundalini awakening. Kundalini will rise higher and higher, because the body is strong and clean. Video demonstrations of all yoga postures mentioned are available online at: http://chakraawakeningbook.com/suite.

Siddhasana, Perfect posture
Chakras: Muladhara, Svadhisthana

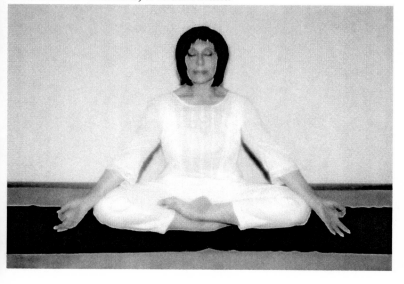

Simhasana, Lion posture
Chakras: Muladhara, Svadhisthana, Manipura

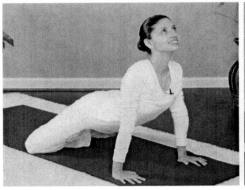
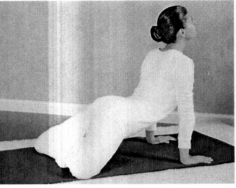

Vrkshasana, Tree posture
Chakras: Muladhara, Ajna, Sahasrara

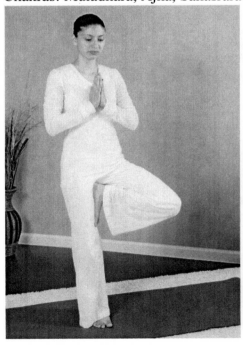
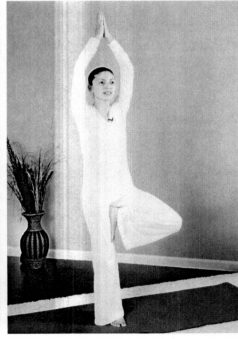

Padmasana, Lotus posture
Chakra: Muladhara

Gomukhasana, Cow-face posture
Chakra: Muladhara

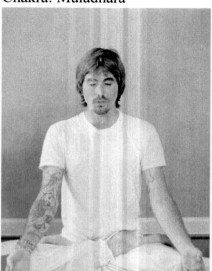

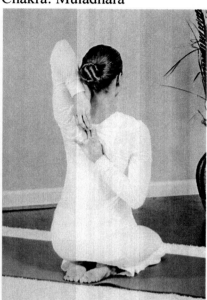

Bhunamanasana, Greeting Earth posture
Chakras: Muladhara, Svadhisthana

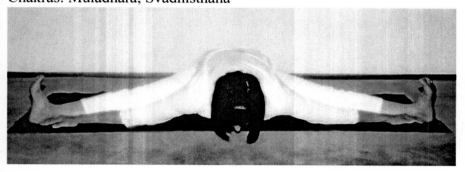

Naukasana, Boat posture
Chakra: Manipura

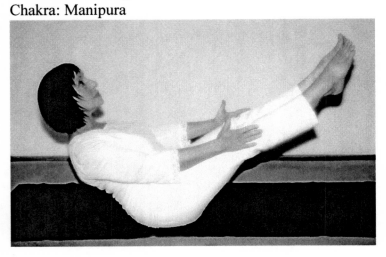

Bhekasana, Frog posture
Chakra: Svadhisthana

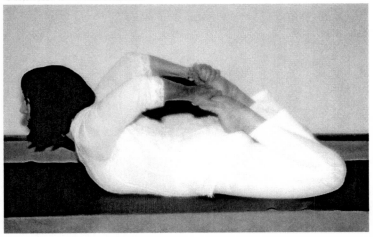

Bhujanghasana, Cobra posture
Chakras: Manipura, Anaahat

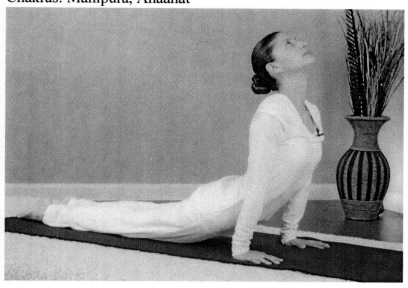

Ustrasana, Camel posture
Chakras: Anaahat, Vishuddhi

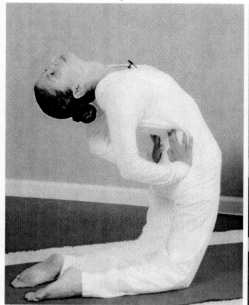 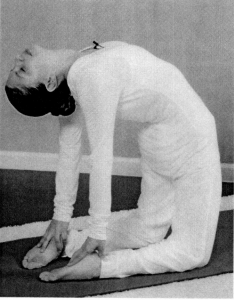

Ardha Matsyendrasana, Half-Fish posture
Chakra: Anaahat

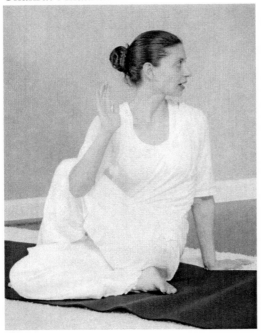

Matsyasana, Full-Fish posture
Chakra: Anaahat

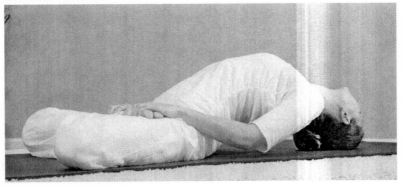

Hastapadasana, Standing Forward-Bend posture
Chakra: Manipura

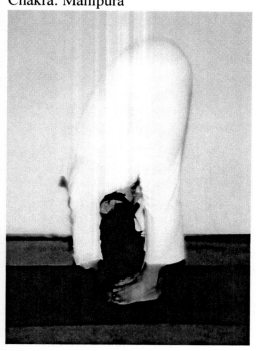

Jnanu Sirsasana, Head-to-Knee posture
Chakra: Vishuddhi

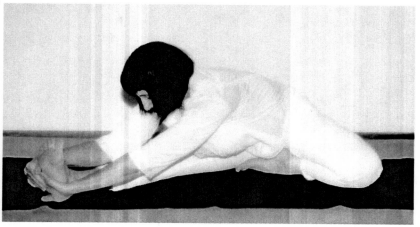

Shalabhasana, Locust posture
Chakra: Vishuddhi

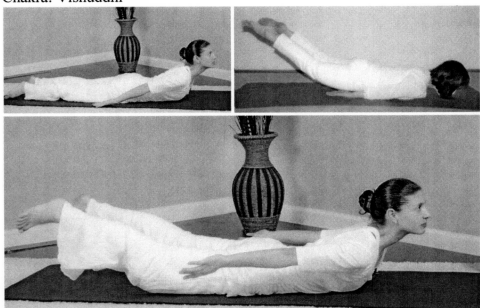

Dandasana, Staff posture
Chakra: Manipura

Goduhasana, Cow-milking posture
Chakra: Muladhara

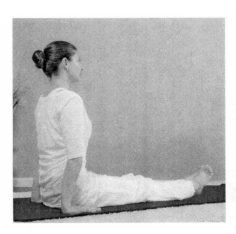

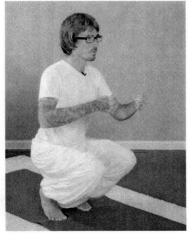

Chakrasana, Wheel posture
Chakras: All seven chakras

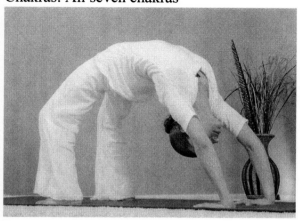

Halasana, Plow posture
Chakra: Vishuddhi

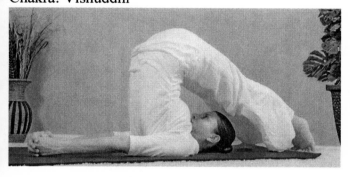

Mayurasana, Peacock posture
Chakra: Manipura

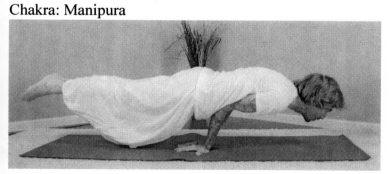

Kurmasana, Tortoise posture *(as taught by Acharya Shree Yogeesh)*
Chakra: Manipura

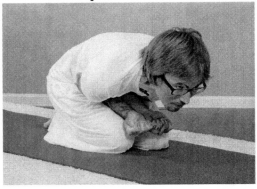

Garudasana, Eagle posture
Chakra: Ajna

Ananda Balasana, Happy Baby posture
Chakra: Ajna

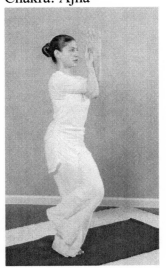

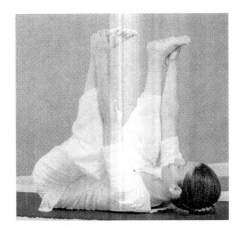

Sirsasana, Headstand posture
Chakra: Ajna

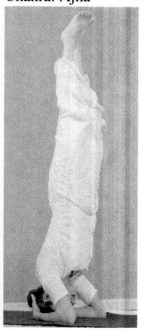

Salamba Sarvangasana, Supported Shoulderstand posture
Chakra: Ajna

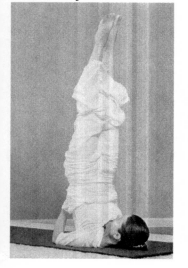

Bhekasana, Frog Posture *(as taught by Acharya Shree Yogeesh)*
Chakra: Svadhisthana

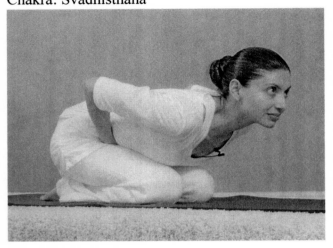

Kurmasana, Tortoise posture
Chakra: Manipura

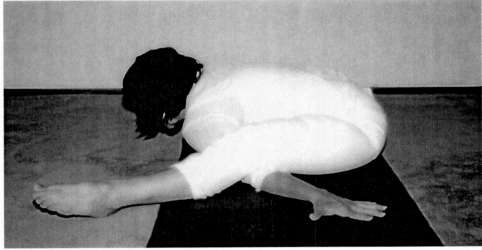

Suryanamaskara, Sun Salutation sequence
Chakra: Manipura

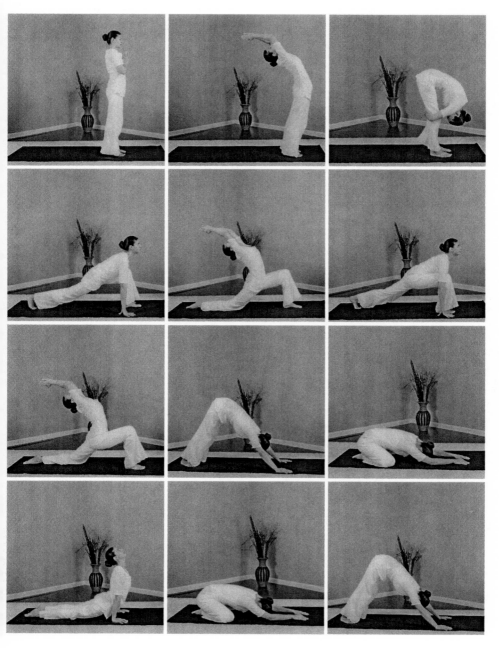

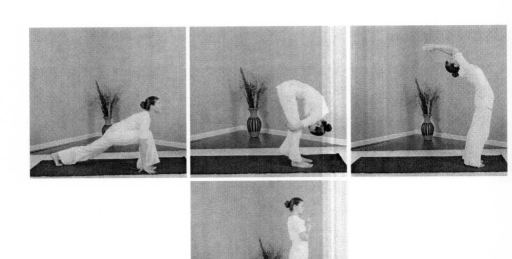

MUDRAS

A *mudra* is like a yoga posture for your hands. You can watch how to perform these mudras at http://chakraawakeningbook.com/suite.

Bhu mudra
Chakra: Muladhara

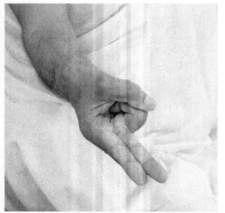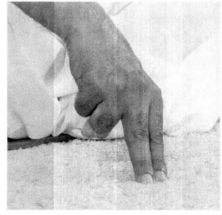

First, roll your ring and pinky fingers into your palm, and cover them by wrapping your thumb over the top. Hold this finger position, and slowly turn your hand so the palm faces the ground. Lightly press the tips of your index and middle fingers to the ground.

Yoni mudra
Chakra: Svadhisthana

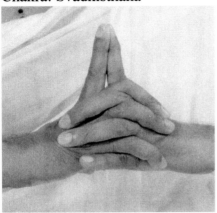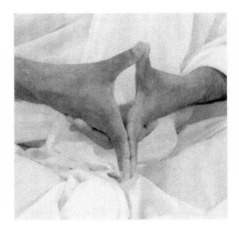

Place your hands together in the "prayer position." Clasp all of your fingers together, except for the index fingers and thumbs. Now turn your hands so the index fingers are pointing toward the ground. Lastly, stretch your thumbs upward and away from your index fingers, and press the roots of your fingers into each other so the palms seperate.

Matangi mudra
Chakra: Manipura

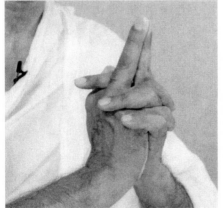

Start by placing your hands in the "prayer postion." Clasp all of your fingers together, except for your middle fingers and thumbs. Lightly press your middle fingers together. Position your thumbs side-by-side, so the knuckles are facing towards you, and they should naturally press against the index finger which is in front.

Padma mudra
Chakra: Anaahat

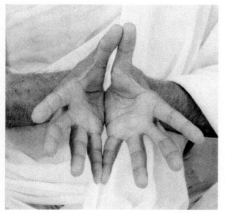 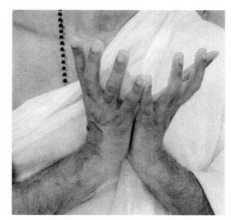

Open your hands by stretching your pinky fingers and thumbs outward. Now touch your thumbs together, and do the same with your pinky fingers. Keep the bottom of your palms touching together. Finally, create the shape of a lotus flower by pushing the lower-palms together, and stretching your knuckles outward. Position this mudra close to your heart.

Shuni mudra
Chakra: Vishuddhi

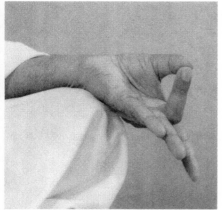

To create the Shuni mudra, simply touch the tip of your thumb with the tip of your middle finger. Extend your other fingers outward.

Jnana mudra
Chakra: Ajna

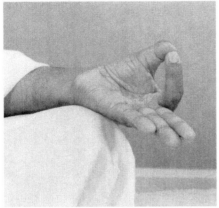

Touch your thumb to the tip of your index finger to create the Jnana mudra. Another mudra which activates and balances the Ajna chakra is the Shanmukhi mudra pranayama; you can find it in the chapter titled, "Pranayama."

Haakini mudra
Chakra: Sahasrara

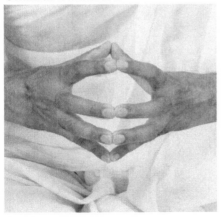 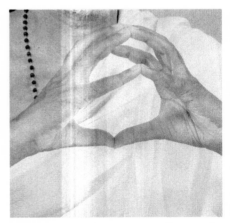

Simply touch all of the fingertips together. No other parts of your hands should be touching.

ABOUT THE AUTHOR

Acharya Shree Yogeesh is a living enlightened master of this era and is the founder of the Siddhayatan Tirth and Spiritual Retreat, a unique 155 acre spiritual pilgrimage site and meditation park in North America providing the perfect atmosphere for spiritual learning, community, and soul awakening to help truth seekers advance spiritually. Acharya Shree is also the founder of the Yogeesh Ashram near Los Angeles, California, Yogeesh Ashram International in New Delhi, India, and the Acharya Yogeesh Primary & Higher Secondary children's school in Haryana, India.

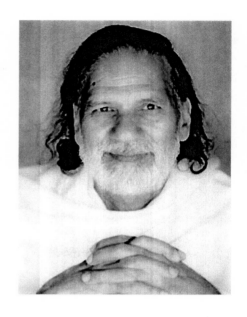

As an inspiring revolutionary spiritual leader and in-demand speaker worldwide, for over forty-five years Acharya Shree has dedicated his life to helping guide hundreds of thousands of people on their spiritual journeys of self-improvement and self-realization. Recently, he was publicly given the highest honor in Agra, India for his spiritual work worldwide, an honor that has never been given by all four Jain sanghs throughout history until now.

It is Acharya Shree's mission to spread the message of nonviolence, vegetarianism, oneness, and total transformation.

Meet him at Siddhayatan.org and FaceBook.com/AcharyaShreeYogeesh.

CONNECT WITH US

Siddhayatan Spiritual Retreat Center

http://siddhayatan.org

Siddhayatan Spiritual Children's Camp

http://spiritualchildrenscamp.com

Acharya Shree Yogeesh's YouTube Channels

http://youtube.com/yogeeshashram

http://youtube.com/siddhayatan

Acharya Shree Yogeesh's Facebook Fan Page

http://facebook.com/AcharyaShreeYogeesh

Awaken Chakras 14-CD course

http://awakenchakras.com

Contact Us

Siddhayatan Tirth
9985 E. Hwy 56
Windom, Texas 75492
info@siddhayatan.org

(903) 487-0717

ACKNOWLEDGMENTS

Thank you to Sadhvi Siddhali Shree, for overseeing and working on this major book project. Your perseverance, tenacity and heart to spread the truth will affect many.

Thanks to -

Miles O'Sullivan, for your help in arranging my discourses into this book. Believe in yourself and your writing talents.

Anubhuti, Cody Deveny, Daniela Romero and Shunta Kobayashi for your help in demonstrating the chakra activation techniques and/or assistance in editing.

Rob Secades, for the book design.
Alannah Avelin, for the bio photo.

CHAKRA AWAKENING
TECHNIQUE SUITE

Get instant access to "How-To" videos so that you can perform the chakra awakening techniques properly and safely as taught by Acharya Shree Yogeesh.

Take full advantage of the unique and special guidance provided in thi suite to help you maximize the benefits of the *Chakra Awakening* techniques.

In the *Chakra Awakening Technique Suite*, you will find:

☑ dynamic and vigorous <u>breathing exercises</u> to purge toxins

☑ effective <u>mudras</u> to create tremendous energy

☑ powerful <u>activation sounds</u> for healing and protection

☑ divine universal <u>mantras</u> never shared before

☑ energetic and chakra activating <u>yoga postures</u>

Learn and master the chakra awakening techniques by watchin the videos and you will feel balanced, grounded, healthie happier and more connected with your higher self.

FOR MORE INFORMATION VISIT:
CHAKRAAWAKENINGBOOK.COM/SUI

SPIRITUAL BOOKS
BY
SIDDHA SANGH PUBLICATIONS

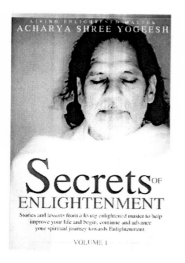

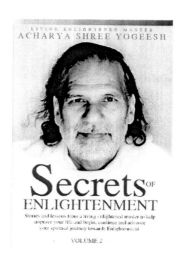

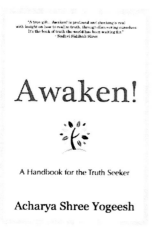

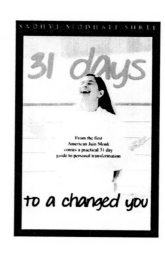